Away from Home
The Mentally Handicapped in Residential Care

By the same author

A mentally handicapped child in the family

MARY McCORMACK

Away from Home

The Mentally Handicapped in Residential Care

CONSTABLE
LONDON

First published in Great Britain 1979
by Constable and Company Limited
10 Orange Street London WC2H 7EG

Hardback ISBN 0 09 462510 7
Paperback ISBN 0 09 463080 1
Set in Monotype Times 10pt
Printed in Great Britain by
The Anchor Press Ltd and bound by
Wm Brendon & Son Ltd both of
Tiptree, Essex

British Library cataloguing in publication data

McCormack, Mary
Away from home
1 Mentally handicapped – Institutional
care – Great Britain
1 Title
362.3′0941 HV3008.G7

For Clare

Contents

Introduction

I suppose every section of society has its cliché. 'What will happen to Johnnie when we're not here to take care of him?' belongs to parents of mentally handicapped children. That or one of its permutations. And it is none the less true for repetition.

It is a problem that starts off as an occasional niggle at the back of your mind when the child is young and builds up, year by unrelenting year, to a constant crescendo of concern. And the concern is not unfounded.

Most mentally handicapped people will spend some of their lives away from home, in residential care. Maybe the biggest part of their lives. At some point, parents are no longer going to be able to continue looking after them at home; or maybe no longer willing to go on making the sacrifices involved. Who, then, will do the job?

The point may not be reached until the parents are old or even till they die. On the other hand, the crisis may come in early childhood or any time in between. Or the family may make the carefully considered decision that, in the child's interests, this is the time to make the break. It depends on the child and on the family, on the amount of support available, on circumstances – on a hundred and one little variables.

Nobody parts lightly with their child, whether that child is five or fifty. No home, hostel or hospital is going to be quite good enough to hypercritical parental eyes, no staff sufficiently devoted. There is no place like home.

The trauma is made even worse by ignorance about the various kinds of residential establishments – on the parents' part and sometimes by the doctors, teachers and social workers who are supposed to be able to help them. The consequent myths that build up about life behind the doors of such places can be more worrying than any reality – and certainly more misleading.

Sadly the professionals and officials in this field do little to dispel the mystique. Maybe they don't even notice it is there. Far from being invited through those closed doors, parents are still viewed with suspicion and occasionally downright dislike in many statutory and non-statutory establishments.

The result is that the first chance many a family gets to look at the possibilities occurs when 'little Johnnie' has already become a crisis case and has to be allocated the first available bed, like it or not. Parent/professional participation, that popular subject of conferences, has not yet reached great heights between families and the people who do now, or will one day soon, be looking after their children.

Parents have a right – and a duty that shouldn't be shirked – to know what is available and to say what they want made available. They also should have a say in their child's future, *the* say – though professionals have been known to disagree with this on the grounds that parents are emotionally involved, dirty words in the mental health service.

Yet, few of us get the opportunity to look inside the various units, other than a brief conducted tour on Open Days, when the residents are out or out of mischief, accompanied by a rosy commentary. This may show you the general taste in wallpaper and whether Matron is a good talker, but it does not answer the real questions.

What would life be like here for *my* son? What sort of people, with what attitudes and ideas would look after him – and how many of them? How would my daughter spend her evenings here? Would she be over-cossetted or under-supervised? What would she eat? Would she be an individual or just another mouth to feed? Would they understand her? Who, as one mother about to part with her daughter put it poignantly, will wipe her nose and kiss her better when she falls down? Who will care? Parents want to know what life is really like there, not what the rule book or the administrator several levels removed from the nursery floor says it should be. They ask about people, too – the kind of people who work in these places and their attitudes to their charges and to their families.

People are so important: far more so than bricks and mortar or suitable settings. If we could design them, some of our problems would be solved. If we can get and keep the right ones from the existing selection, that won't be too bad!

You cannot know what you want for your child if you do not know what exists or is possible. This book then, sets out to provide some of the answers by looking at a random selection of residential establishments, statutory and non-statutory, catering for a variety of ages and degrees of handicap. They are typical of the range available, though obviously every place is different.

My role has been that of a non-participating observer, dropping in at different times, on several visits of varying duration. It is a role open to criticism, too – anyone sitting around my home or yours would be likely to see some things they did not approve off. Nor is it always easy. You may try to be the fly on the wall, but your presence may still alter the behaviour of some people and irritate others. I did not set out to demolish (that path has been trodden efficiently before), to praise, or to produce a pile of neatly recorded statistics. The idea was simply to report and record, as objectively as possible, allowing that all reporting is a little subjective. The viewpoint is that of reporter and parent. One hospital administrator, turning down my request to attach myself to one of the wards (only hospitals were reluctant), gave as a reason that I might 'see things differently' from someone who had experience of working in a residential setting. Differently, yes. More clearly, I hope.

I am grateful to the staff, at all levels, of the various establishments, for their tolerance and co-operation – even if, in some cases, we did see things differently. Grateful, too, to the residents who, when they were capable of welcoming and helping, invariably did so.

In a way, the book was a quest. As the mother of a multiply-handicapped boy now in his teens, I have the same fears and the same need to know the future prospects as every other parent. On that score it was depressing. My research simply reinforced what I suspected – that the more handicapped an individual is, the gloomier the outlook.

For the brighter, more rewarding children and adults there are possibilities opening up. But for those who cannot contribute anything concrete, for the profoundly handicapped who need total care, and for their opposite number – the euphemistically labelled 'behaviour problems' at their destructive worst – there is not a glimmer of light on the horizon. Away from home, their lives are painfully limited and emotionally destitute.

They get no choices. Little inventiveness goes into thinking up ways of improving their lot – little in the way of resources, either. When new ideas of care emerge, the most handicapped are automatically excluded. They take so much time and energy, so much money – and give so little back. They would only rock the boat.

It is easy to forget, when you are writing about the quality of care, that the quantity is desperately short, too. Almost all the residential homes and hospitals – good, bad or indifferent – have waiting lists. Parents at the end of their tether are sometimes grateful for any offer.

Even so, the greatest shortage of places is for the most handicapped children and adults; except for hospital beds, these are practically non-existent. Yet these are the people who are going to need residential care earlier, not least because less help by way of community facilities comes their way, too, when they are living at home. These are the people who need help urgently. They will not go away just because we ignore them.

1

History

In the beginning there was Bethlem, or 'Bedlam', the London hospital for 'idiots and lunatics' that gave the English language a colourful new word. That was in use from 1377 and housed both the mentally ill and the mentally handicapped, because no distinction was made between the two until well into the nineteenth century. Medical treatment in Bethlem, according to reports dated 1815, consisted of purges, bleeding and 'taking the vomits' and inmates were kept chained to the wall, nearly naked, on straw bedding. Until 1770, visitors paid a penny a time to come in and laugh at their antics.

Things were not much better in the other institutions to which the mentally handicapped found their way around this time. 'Pauper lunatics' were confined to the workhouse; others were in prison – insanity or handicap being no excuse for crime. Wealthier families sometimes had their mentally handicapped relatives committed to private madhouses, run for profit and with only nominal inspection. The rest lived at home – locked in the proverbial shuttered rooms of large houses to hide the family's shame, or tied up in a corner by poorer families, to stop them bothering the neighbours.

The first glimmer of hope came in 1792, with the York Retreat. Its founder, the Quaker, William Tuke, evolved humanitarian methods of treatment that were unheard of then, and which we still accept now – no unnecessary drugs, no restraint, but keeping patients occupied and taking them out to 'tea parties and religious meetings'. It was private, it catered for only thirty people and none of them poor (servants could be accommodated for eight to fifteen shillings a week!) but it showed what could be achieved, and Tuke's writings shook up public consciousness. A series of reforms followed and County Asylums began to spring up. By 1881, there were 29,452 people diagnosed as mentally handicapped in public institutions, only three per cent of these in places specifically designed for them.

The first colony for the mentally handicapped was set up at the turn of the century 'for life-long segregation and permanent care'. Here, at the Sandlebridge Colony, 170 male and 116 female patients of all ages lived self-sufficiently, cut off from the community, with their own school, hospital and farm. It was a model to be widely copied before it lost favour. It is not hard to see today's village communities as new, improved versions of the old idea; and some staff within hospitals would like to see them develop along the lines of sheltered communities for the severely handicapped.

At the time of the original colonies however, the main concern was not for the comfort of the handicapped people. It was more to do with the widespread fears of them breeding and lowering the intellectual tone of the nation. Segregation meant safety – for the normal community.

In 1914 there were thirty-eight institutions exclusively for the mentally handicapped, and several small homes run by church societies and welfare groups. The voluntary sector was getting a foothold. Four years later, despite the war turning people's thoughts to other matters, there were forty-eight local voluntary associations registered.

The Wood Committee of 1929 insisted that institutions should 'not be a stagnant pool but a flowing lake'. It suggested the provision of schools and workshops to prepare patients for life outside and half-way houses or hostels where the more capable handicapped could live under supervision and go out to work. Hospitals started sending patients out to work. Occupation centres opened and, with them, a few hostels.

It was a small swing towards community care. Since 1913 Local Authorities had held responsibility for making provision for people in their area. In 1948, with the introduction of the Welfare State, responsibility for institutions was transferred to the new hospital authorities.

By the mid-Fifties, there had been no major reforms for over sixty years and hospitals had fallen into an appalling state. There was over-crowding, under-staffing and a desperate shortage of finance to do anything about life in these decaying Victorian monuments.

The 1959 Mental Health Act was the start of a new era of reform. Suddenly doors were open and throughout the next decade people seemed to be flocking into hospitals in droves to see and report for themselves – politicians, working parties, sociologists, journalists.

Enoch Powell, then Minister for Health, announced plans to get rid of thousands of hospital beds, starting a controversy that still rages. Books, such as Pauline Morris's *Put Away*, highlighted the dreadful conditions to be found in some wards. Reports of cruelty and misconduct in specific hospitals made newspaper headlines.

In 1969 and 1970, the late Richard Crossman, as Secretary of State for Health, set out on his own voyage of discovery around the hospitals. He found shortages of money, staff, beds, space – and painfully low morale. As a result, he launched a minimum standards exercise, with a list of specific objectives, like not allowing more than fifty adults or thirty children to a ward and providing personal clothing for each person instead of a communal wardrobe.

The great guiding light of our time was the government White Paper *Better Services for the Mentally Handicapped*, published in 1971. It was a comprehensive document covering many aspects of the lives of mentally handicapped people, but its most publicized proposal was the move from hospital to community care.

The mentally handicapped were to go into the community, living at home where at all possible. Where not, Local Authorities were to step up the provision of small, local homes and hostels, and hospitals were to send their residents out to these. Children were no longer to be admitted to hospital or kept there, unless their needs could not be met anywhere else.

But saying what should be done is one thing, implementing it another. Definitions were vague, deadlines were not set. The movement has been slower than hoped. The small community homes on everyone's doorstep are still a pipe-dream.

The National Development Group for the Mentally Handicapped* was set up in 1975 to monitor services and advise the government on policy. It has kept the ball rolling, producing a series of clear-cut pamphlets, filled with common sense conclusions and suggestions.

We have come a long way from Bedlam. We still have a long way to go.

*The National Development Group for the Mentally Handicapped, Alexander Fleming House, London SE1 6BY.

2

The Health Service – Something Old, Something New

Hospitals are not merely buildings any more: they are big, emotive issues. They have been since the White Paper of 1971, *Better Services for the Mentally Handicapped*, instigated a move from institutional to community care, from provision by the Department of Health to that by Local Authorities.

Though hospitals are still the biggest providers of residential care, the great exodus has reduced the number of residents nationally from nearly 60,000 to 50,000 so far, halving the bed count in some wards. It is still going on – and so, too, are the battles between various professions, verbally at least, that the move engendered, as well as the confusion of who will do what for whom in the future.

There are people – parents and professionals – who want hospitals closed completely, irrespective of where Local Authorities will find the money to cope with patients left on their hands and those yet to come.

Others – including not unnaturally those who work in them – believe that hospitals can adapt to modern ideas and still offer many of the handicapped the best possible care. They do not accept that all mentally handicapped people are happier in the community – the hospital itself is a community, after all.

What appears to be happening, though it is hard to see clearly through the highly charged aura that surrounds the issue, is that hospitals are staying put, but adapting rapidly – to different ideas of care and often different people. They are opening doors wide, inviting volunteers in, taking residents out more, providing training courses that may lead to more independent living, involving themselves more with the mentally handicapped living outside the hospital walls. Specialist hospital staff, like psychologists, doctors and nurses, are increasingly spending more time working in the community, working, sometimes in prickly harmony, alongside Social Services.

Most interesting, perhaps, hospital policy-makers are experimenting with alternative types of residential care: typically small satellite homes like the two featured in this section. First in this field and ahead of the hullabaloo was the Wessex Regional Health Authority, which opened two community hostels for children in the late Sixties.

The children's units and the adults' hostels which followed were masterminded by Dr Albert Kushlick, who had to fight hard to get people to listen to his wildly radical notion that mentally handicapped people could live fuller, happier lives in a home-like environment, cared for by people who were not necessarily nurses.

The Wessex Experiment, as it became known, is still being monitored and analysed in detail by Dr Kushlick and his staff, so that other people covering the same ground can learn from their mistakes and successes.

All hospitals now train residents in areas that should enable them to move on to a more independent, community life – people they might not have considered candidates for such a place a few years back. Private lodging houses, the old standby for ex-patients being discharged, have had a deservedly bad press, and hostels are now the main aim. But there are not enough of those to go round.

The hardest thing to change is the attitude of people who have worked a life-time in hospitals. Many observers, including voluntary societies for the mentally handicapped, insist that they will never be acceptable until the medical domination has been removed and they are no longer the preserves of doctors and nurses, but homely places run by a new, non-medical profession.

At the end of 1978, on the premise that whatever White Papers advised, there would still be people living in large hospitals for many years to come, the National Development Group for the Mentally Handicapped (NDG) produced a report on *Helping Mentally Handicapped People in Hospital.* The Group makes no bones about its view that there should be a more radical shift to community care than envisaged in 1971. Meanwhile, certain improvements should be made immediately to make life better for the 50,000 hospital residents, 4,000 of them children.

It is suggested that (a) life in hospital should be more home-like, reducing living units to a maximum of six places for children and twelve for adults; (b) there should be full assessment and a training programme for each resident, plus a hospital training team to take responsibility for all training activities; (c) there should be better training for staff involved with children – heads of all children's units should have a qualification in child care – and there should be more of them; and (d) there should be improved health care and specialist services. One of the surprises – or shocks – was that hospital residents often get poorer primary health services and less access to specialists than their counterparts in the community, due to staff shortages and lack of information.

The Group found that hospitals vary tremendously, as do wards within individual hospitals; that some places have improved greatly in the past decade and some hardly at all. They blame not only the obvious shortages of staff and resources, but 'inertia'.

What does the hopefully influential NDG suggest? 'They key to a better service lies in making each individual hospital more accountable to residents' families and to the public at large.' And so say all of us! But the Group goes further and sets out details of a monitoring system that could be used at all levels to make this a reality.

The Hospital

There are no gates to the hospital. You can drive in one side, off a main road, and out the other into small-town suburbia, covering a mile of minor road and hospital tarmac in-between. It grew, like all the hospitals of its time, in isolation. It is still now surrounded by acres of grounds and good arable farm land, but through the trees you can see the high-rise windows of an overspill new town nearby.

The big house that became the administrative offices was a family home when it was built a hundred years ago. In the days when the rich were richer, this was the Hall, the local squire's pad. Inside the door is a large square reception hall, with doors opening off it and a wide staircase. There is an open fireplace and a portrait of a late consultant psychiatrist above. It still looks an unlikely base for nursing offices, administrators and switchboard operators.

The Hall became a hospital for the mentally handicapped in the Thirties and, over the years, wards, workshops, and prefabs have sprouted up around it in apparent architectural disorder, like chess pieces moved by a manic player. If there was rhyme or reason for the layout at the time, it is no longer obvious to an outsider. Not that it matters much except from an aesthetic viewpoint. It functions. Layout is the least of the hospital's problems.

It is one of four mental handicap hospitals in a group controlled by an Area Health Authority. Some facilities, including laundry and the school its ten children attend, are at the nearby sister hospital, which does not please everyone. Altogether, there are 293 residents and an interim secure unit is near completion and will take disturbed patients with the aim of training them back to the community.

Community care, in its variable forms, has taken back many of the higher grade residents over the past few years. The numbers used to be double, and older nurses tell you of being in charge of seventy patients in a ward with only one helper.

'It was just custodial care,' one said. 'We used to joke that epileptic patients never fall on the floor. The beds were too close together to find the space.' There is a hint almost of nostalgia for the bad old days.

Things are changing, have been for the past ten years. Hospitals are in a constant state of flux and this makes it difficult to assess them. What exists now may be quite different in five years' time.

With more able patients gone out, nurses have had to learn to care for a population made up almost entirely of the severely and multiply handicapped and the disturbed – without the balancing effect and the practical help of the old-style 'better' patients.

They still haven't quite got the hang of it. Workshops (assembly work and packing the inevitable curlers) are fine for patients who can use them. There is even an incentive scheme – they earn more for good behaviour and hard work. Recreational facilities – table tennis, cards, disco, games with other hospitals, evening outings – are fun for the more able. But as one nurse, working with the heavily handicapped, put it, 'Only the presentable-looking ones go on these things, not our lot'.

Most of her patients indeed would get little pleasure from such outings. The clever bit is finding something they could join in and enjoy and this I suspect is going to take not only more expert consideration, but a far higher staff ratio. It has to be done, because if hospitals go their predicted route, they will soon end up with only these very difficult people and they won't know what to do with them.

'We will have to change as our patients change. We are all aware of that,' said a nursing officer.

'However handicapped they are, they have a right to their entertainment,' said a nursing assistant helping with recreation. What did she do in this way for multiply handicapped Sally? 'I can read to her. She can listen to the music and be pushed around in her chair in a little dance with the others.'

But inside the recreation hall the music was deafening, and Sally, sitting in the middle of the room in a wheelchair and used to only the sound of quiet voices on her ward, was crying.

It is easy to knock hospitals. With their rigid routines, institutional air and their notorious staff shortages, they are the 'Aunt Sallies' of the Health Service. They cannot be choosy about patients. They have to take those referred, often the biggest problems. In the past ten years they have been criticized unmercifully by press, public, parents and other professionals. Before you condemn, though, you should know the problems.

'The public were up in arms about conditions in hospitals. They were partly responsible for us opening hostels and group homes and sending patients out to live in the community,' said a nursing officer. 'Yet you should see the fuss made by these good people when we try to open a hostel in their road.'

This had happened just before I began visiting the hospital. Local residents were fighting tooth and nail to stop a group of patients living in a house in their neighbourhood, on the grounds that they would be a danger to their children.

An invitation to visit the hospital and meet these 'dangerous' people was refused. No point in letting the facts spoil a good prejudice.

'The worst thing to me was that the objectors were not old people set in their ways,' a nurse told me, 'but young couples in their twenties and thirties, who you would expect to know better.'

If I were a subnormality hospital nurse, I would be pretty paranoid at the public vision of me as an uncaring monster not far removed from the custodial keepers of Bedlam. They have, due to a few cases of cruelty and malpractice brought against a tiny minority, had a very bad press.

From nursing assistant (possibly the most important person in terms of their child's care, to a parent) to nursing officer, I found them practical, caring and aware people. It cannot be that easy for the older, senior staff (there are too few young people in the higher echelons) to accept and encourage a barrage of constantly changing new ideas. They have had to. It's just that the cogs of such a big organization take so long to turn, they may not be there to see them implemented.

If there is a general staff attitude strikingly different from people working in small homes, it is their acceptance of themselves as professional people doing a job they like for a wage, rather than dedicated folks with a vocation. 'I'm not dedicated. I believe we do a good job and should get paid for it. I'm here mainly because I enjoy the job. If I didn't I would leave.'

'What qualities do you look for?' I asked a nurse-tutor who takes on students for the three-year RNMS (Registered Nurse for the Mentally Subnormal) course run at the hospital.

'I don't know,' he admitted. 'It's just a gut feeling that they are right. Nothing much to do with academic qualifications, although we are getting more highly educated people nowadays, and younger ones. At one time it was rare to have anyone under twenty-five apply. I would be more inclined to take someone who said he needed the job – because that's why I became a nurse – than someone who talked about wanting to help people. I'm interested in passing on attitudes as much as skills. More so. That's the main reason I teach.'

This man had trained as both a general and mental nurse. So had some of the other senior staff and a few were State Registered Nurses who accidentally found themselves involved in this branch of nursing.

'I had young children and we had bought a house in this area. I couldn't travel a long distance and this was the only job available. I was terrified. I didn't know what to expect or how long I would stay', said a woman who has been there for twenty-five years. People either leave quickly, they say – or stay and stay.

There are calls from many quarters for a new profession to care for the mentally handicapped, arguing that they are not ill and do not, therefore, need nurses. This inspires hostility from the nurses, understandably as a threat to their jobs and status, but also 'because it will be a lower-paid profession and attract "pin money" workers, rather than long-term professionals. This will bring down the standard of care,' argued a student nurse.

Almost everyone I talked to had strong opinions and good ideas – parent/nurse associations to encourage parent participation, talks by professionals for parents at the hospital, talks by parents for nurses in training, using the hospital as a community care base with lots more short-term, overnight and crêche facilities.

This last suggestion seems impractical in view of where the hospital is situated, but several of the staff were convinced that the hospital, not the Social Services, was the peg on which community care should be hung. Said one: 'We have the experience – it is a very specialist field and I am not convinced the Social Services have the expertise to deal with the mentally handicapped. We have the facilities here. The community, the people in general, do not accept our patients. They just see the ugliness or the peculiar behaviour. We don't notice that. We see the individual underneath.'

Either way, the bulk of the ideas are probably doomed to die before they find their way up the long ladder to the people who can do something about them. At the top of the hospital tree sit the administrator, a consultant psychiatrist (plus normally a second psychiatrist, but that position was vacant when I was visiting the hospital) and a senior nursing officer. There are five other nursing officers – three responsible for a group of wards each, one on night duty, one over recreation and work centres and another responsible for rehabilitation.

There is also a psychology department, the mention of which is accompanied by much raising of eyebrows and an explanation from a young nurse: 'They are not very interested in *my* patients'.

It is a rigid pecking order. A part-time nursing assistant calling in to tell the administrator or senior consultant what she would like to see done, is inconceivable – although it was pointed out to me on numerous occasions that, compared with any other kind of hospital, relationships between different staff levels are strikingly informal. It is, I suppose, relative.

HONEYSUCKLE WARD – MULTIPLY HANDICAPPED ADULTS

Tuesday 9.30 a.m.

The 'babies' of Honeysuckle Ward are being bathed, changed and dressed for the day. This morning routine has been going on since 8 a.m., when the day staff came on duty and started the ball rolling by feeding the 'babies', still lying in their cots. Then, one by one, they are lifted on to a trolley, their nappies and nightclothes removed, wheeled into the bathroom for their morning dip, taken back out to their room, dressed and placed in a wheelchair.

It takes two nursing assistants, working together, to do each job, because the 'babies', as everyone involved with the ward calls them, are in fact five physically/mentally handicapped teenagers of eighteen-plus and one thirty-three-year-old man.

They are relative newcomers to the hospital. Colin, the thirty-three-year-old, arrived from another hospital four years ago. He is so frail that one of the women assistants can lift him in her arms and carry him to the bathroom – and so distorted from the waist down by spasticity that he cannot sit in a wheelchair. Consequently, his world is one room. 'He's never been further away than that tree,' said one of the two domestics, pointing to a tree on the grassy patch outside the ward. 'Sometimes someone will carry him out on a hot day. He enjoys that.'

Colin enjoys everything that brings people near him. He sits all day on a giant bean bag on the floor in a corner of the room – his only alternative position is lying in his cot – and watches people pass by and smiles if you look his way. Often he clutches a big rag doll his mother brought him. Only he and Roddy, the other male patient, see their parents regularly; but Colin's mother, a widow with another handicapped son, is finding it difficult to get over to see him as often as she did.

'Fancy a great big boy like you playing with a dolly. You should be ashamed of yourself,' another of the domestic staff stopped to say, and he beamed. 'He watches everything,' someone said. 'He can see into the corridor through that window. I bet he would tell some tales if he could talk.'

In fact Colin's life on a giant bean bag has little in it to talk about. Except for those rare excursions out on to the grass, every hour of it is passed in a small, tidy, scrupulously clean room that makes up a third of the sleeping accommodation of Honeysuckle Ward.

There are two other wards or small dormitories, plus a kitchen where the ward's food is cooked, a dining-room and a day room with television. Honeysuckle is home to twenty-four patients, with two beds to spare for emergencies – all male except for the four physically handicapped girls. Many of them are elderly, not well or there temporarily after illness or an operation, before returning to a more active, noisy ward. A couple are blind. It functions in a limited capacity as a sick bay.

Most of the patients are low-grade and not capable of going to the hospital workshops during the day – even if they were well enough. Some incontinent men have to be bathed up to three times a day. 'Easier than trying to wash them down,' one of the nursing assistants explained.

Not the liveliest place in the world, by any means, but at least the bulk of the patients have the freedom to walk from room to room, to go outside as they please, to go over to the recreation hall.

For Colin, there are no such privileges and the sad thing is that he would probably enjoy them more than most. It is more convenient to keep the physically handicapped all together in one place. At one time he used to be carried, with his bean bag, into the sitting-room to watch television or see the world go by.

When the 'babies' arrived a year ago, from another children's hospital, the ward and the routine had to be rearranged to accommodate them. It was plainly difficult to find a place to put them. There are other physically handicapped patients in the hospital, a few on each ward, but none so helpless as the newcomers. There had to be ground-floor accommodation and adequate bathing facilities to hand. The nursing officer in charge of the ward is concerned and caring. She worries about them, about their comfort and their safety. 'I know it is not the ideal place to have four teenage girls in a ward full of men, but their room is out-of-bounds to all other patients. We let nobody else in.'

A nursing assistant echoes this. 'There are male patients in the hospital – though not in this ward, I don't think – who definitely would take advantage of them. We can't mix them up more with the other patients. You can't be changing and dressing them in front of those old men.' But can't they eat with them, sit in the dayroom with them? No – the dining-room is overcrowded already and there is no space for wheelchairs. Taking the 'babies' into the common room has been tried and caused problems. 'They make a lot of noise, baby sounds. The old men don't like it and you have to consider them, too. It has made their lives more inconvenient since these arrived. They have less attention. If you try to put any of the "babies" down on the floor by the television, Patrick [one of the patients who uses a wheelchair] will run them down, or one man who is blind will walk on them. Any of the others can stumble into them, they don't always look where they are going.'

So the 'babies' stay put, though each one, excluding Colin, has his or her own wheelchair and is sometimes taken across to the recreation hall for a couple of hours in the morning or out for a push on a warm day. There was no outing the morning I was there. The 'rec' nurse (two nursing assistants working in shifts are in charge of the day and evening activities in the recreation hall) is taking a group out in the grounds to do yoga. The 'babies' can hardly join in that so, one by one, they are dressed and nappied. Muzak melodies float in the air. Two of the girls wear baggy bottle-green crimplene cat-suits – really awful things, and each of them has an identical one; but the nursing officer has gone to great lengths to get these made and I know, personally, the difficulty of getting an all-in-one garment this size.

Underneath her cat-suit, Sally, whom I have seen being dressed, wears a vest with holes in it and a tea-stained (though freshly laundered) T-shirt. All wear is specially made, including fur-lined soft boots costing £15 a pair. Does it matter? Are these little touches important? I don't know – but parents care. One of the nursing assistants on Honeysuckle mentioned that Roddy's mother, who visits regularly, is very fussy about what he wears.

A nurse on another ward told me, with some irritation: 'Parents never ask me what drugs their children are having or about their behaviour. The only questions they ask are why a girl is not wearing tights or why her hair is not cut in the style they like. It is all-important that they look presentable, whatever else happens.'

This row of inanimate teenagers – for someone with a mentally/physically handicapped child who may need hospital care – is incredibly depressing. All looking blankly ahead at a wall and a row of cots or with heads hanging down, seeing nothing. There is a sense of hopelessness, a feeling that everyone has given up on the 'babies'.

'What else *can* you do for them?' one woman asks, and you begin to think she is right. Certainly with no time and no specialist information, *she* can't do more.

But why weren't the four girls and Roddy down on the floor or on playmats or play cushions – with toys and mobility aids, moving in whatever fashion their spasticity will allow, finding some tiny bit of stimulation? 'They can't move, they can't play, they only lie there,' explained another woman. And they never will move, given no chance to try.

The cots, with their cupboards beside each one, take up three-quarters of the room, so there is very little floor space for physical activities. It was originally a four-bedded room but, with the chairs moved out, it is usable.

'I'd like to have another room we could put them in during the day, to make a change from them being in their bedroom,' said one nursing assistant with some imagination, though she was only thinking of putting them out there in their chairs. 'I don't know if it would make any difference to them, but I would feel better about it.'

They are, I was told, put down sometimes in the afternoon. 'But it is too much of a nuisance. They bang their elbows and it is surprising how far they move.' They never see a physiotherapist, because the hospital cannot get one. 'In any case, what would they do for these little ones?' said a nurse – and when I suggested they might give the ward staff tips on ways to help the children, she pointed out that nobody would be happy with nurses taking over physiotherapists' jobs.

A nursing assistant put it more succinctly. 'Look, what would be the point of me wondering if I could teach Lucy to crawl? I don't have the time to stop and think about it, let alone the time to teach her.' 'What would you most like to see changed?' I asked one woman, expecting something on the lines of 'More time to be with the patients.' 'The laundry arrangements,' she said, predictably perhaps, heaving sheets off a bed and putting new ones on. 'We are always short. The children's ward has its own washing-machine. They get more perks. It would make a great difference if we had one here.' Later, the nursing officer pointed out reasonably that there would not be time for them to do laundry – unless an extra person, a housekeeper, was employed.

At 11 a.m. the patients are in their day positions, the beds are made and it is time for a tea break. 'Time to collapse' one nurse put it – and, indeed, they have worked non-stop and incredibly hard. In two pairs (one SEN among them in charge), they have seen to feeding, changing, bathing (or washing – baths for the abler men are on a rota), shaving where necessary and dressing twenty-four patients.

'It is the heaviest ward in the hospital,' Paula, who has been a nursing assistant for two years, said. 'I don't think extra staff would help, though. You just get in each other's way. We only have two baths and it gets crowded. You just have to have a tight routine worked out.' Wouldn't this job be easier for men? 'We've had men, Paula said. 'They make great charge nurses, but when it comes to hard work, the women still seem to end up doing it.'

They make their own tea and collapse as predicted around a table in the day room. Some of the men wander around or sit aimlessly. The 'babies' in the back room have been left there, but there are domestics in and out.

Nursing assistants are a vital part of the running of a subnormality hospital. They are right at grass roots, working closely with the patients and for the least reward. They are under-rated and rarely consulted – though the nursing officer insists that trained ward staff are instructed to discuss cases with them at weekly meetings. The assistants themselves don't seem aware of it.

'They never ask us to conferences,' one of them said. 'I think they should. I hear somebody is trying to get us included. I mean, if one of these kids spoke or seemed ill or anything, we are the ones who would notice. It might be ages before one of the trained nurses spotted it.'

They are – the ones I met – hard-working, pleasant and sensible; but they do what they are told, what the system and the hierarchy dictates. 'Let's face it,' one of them said, 'we do the job for the money, but there are easier ways of earning more.'

They come from all sorts of diverse occupations – shops, offices, part-time collecting and delivering, domestic work – rarely anything connected with the mentally handicapped. Mostly they live locally and have children at school or grown up. Men rarely apply for such jobs and when they do and are accepted, they tend to be directed towards night duty.

The nursing officer likes to have a proportion of women who have brought up children of their own. 'They have experience to fall back on. They are homely and understanding.'

One of the nursing assistants bears this out. 'This ward is like living with a house full of kids. To be honest, the first few times I had to change nappies on adults, I did gag a bit, but I'd done it with my own kids, so it wasn't so much of a shock as it would be to a young girl. You get used to it very quickly.'

Far more than with the teenage house-mother in the small homes, I would feel confident leaving my child in the care of most of them for a short while. What they do lack is imagination. It is not encouraged here – there isn't time and it isn't convenient.

Paula had been on an in-service training course, spread over twelve weeks, but the chance only came after she had been there for two years. It would have helped at the outset. New recruits have to learn as they go along. 'I learned to do all the things I'd been doing already,' she said wryly. 'We are taught about stimulating the patients, but when is there time?'

Emotion is out too. One nursing assistant used to pass the Children's Ward each day on the way to her own job, and regularly saw a little girl crying in the doorway.

'I used to go on duty in tears myself every morning. The nursing officer told me to go into the Children's Ward and keep going in until it did not affect me. You can't work if you feel that much for them all the time.'

They do talk to their 'babies', tickling them and teasing them as they change nappies and bath them. Apart from that, they say, they have no time to spend with them. If they finish a few minutes early, they are expected to go and help with the older men.

It is not always the shortage of staff that is the problem in hospitals, but how existing staff are used, the obsession with caring for the furniture and fittings even before the patients' needs. It is easier to make a bed than attempt to stimulate an unresponsive person; easier not to question routine.

'Ours not to reason why,' said one of the nursing assistants, summing it up perfectly, when she was told Sally could not be taken over to the 'rec' after all. She pushed her in beside the others, put a tambourine (the only toy she likes) in her hand and carried on with the next task.

Despite this very limited amount of attention, the five most recent arrivals have made progress. Sally will say her name, because she has heard the nurses repeat it often. Another girl calls out the names of some of the nurses.

But they have little enough chance to learn nurses' names. The policy of the hospital is for staff to move around frequently. This is partly, I was told, to present them with new challenges and stop them becoming complacent. It also ensures that they do not become too attached to a particular patient or group, an occupational hazard with women working on the Children's Ward. A domestic who has been on Honeysuckle for years said she would not do nursing because of this. 'They don't move us around. I wouldn't want to change. The ward gets like a family to you.'

The nursing assistants laughed at the suggestion that they could ask to stay on whichever ward they fancied. 'Sometimes you are left for months, even years in the one place, but that is unusual,' one said. 'I should think the sure way not to get put on a ward you like is to ask!'

It seems unfair – and again unimaginative – to remove this one bit of continuity from the lives of patients so handicapped. When the only faces you see are those washing and feeding you and hopefully smiling at you, what does it do to your security when they disappear suddenly to be replaced by unfamiliar people?

Some of the staff themselves agree, though not necessarily for the same reason. 'Changing people round for the sake of it is pointless,' said a fairly cynical male charge nurse from another ward. 'Nobody is good at everything. Some people are good with children, some with the profoundly handicapped, some with disturbed patients. They should be left where they fit.'

It seems a fair point. Even at the risk of familiarity breeding institutionalization in staff, a charge levelled regularly at subnormality hospital nurses, there is a lot to be said for keeping square pegs out of round holes.

It is approaching midday when the cigarettes are put away and the tea cups taken back to the kitchen. For the full-timers it is a long day, twelve hours straight through, three days on, then three off. 'You come in here first thing in the morning and it is night when you go out. After a couple of days, you forget there is anything else in life. It is a little world of its own.'

The 'babies'' midday happening is about to start. One feeding/changing session runs into another. At midday they will be fed their lunches, still in their chairs. It is generally meat and two veg – whatever the rest of the ward has, they get minced up. Plus a sweet and a cup of tea to follow, in a beaker with a spout. They drink a lot of tea. A cup from the night-nurse when nappies are changed at around 7 a.m. before the day people come on. Another with breakfast, a cup at 3 p.m. and more after the evening meal. It was quite an event to see staff remember to give regular drinks to people who could not ask for them.

Thursday 5.45 p.m.

Tea is nearly over. It takes half to three-quarters of an hour to feed the 'babies' two courses and their cup of tea in their cots. They are not difficult to feed. 'They open their mouths happily for any food. They look very excited when they see it coming,' one of the two nursing assistants (a full-timer and part-timer) said. They are amazingly placid patients.

Years of living in homes and hospitals have got rid of any faddiness and, besides, meal times are the big events of the day, bringing attention. Only Colin retains a bit of independent spirit. He will not eat eggs.

Watching Jill feeding Lucy is a bit alarming. The girl, dark, pretty and painfully thin, lies flat on her back as the fruit and cream is spooned in. There is no choking, no problem. She chews and swallows it easily. Her minced pork pie has gone with the same ease and so does her cup of tea.

All the girls are wearing dresses and stretch pants which are too small and too stretched and tend to be nearer their knees. Nevertheless, they look much better and happier than the last time I saw them. They have been in their cots since after lunch, the usual arrangement.

'They are ready for a lie-down after the morning in their chairs,' one nurse said. 'They don't like long stretches in their chairs.'

It has been a more eventful day than usual. They all went over to the recreation hall, where enough ambulant and responsible patients were found to take them for a walk in the grounds. There is never any question of the staff on the wards taking them out. Two is the maximum number dealing with them at one time – not much good for five chairs.

Besides, one pointed out, she would not like to hand the responsibility for them over to another patient. 'They might walk out down the drive and disappear or leave them somewhere and forget about them. Like a young child would with a toy.'

'You don't get the quality of patient you used to,' she said seriously – then laughed as the ridiculousness of the statement sunk in. But she is right. It was easier when there were patients capable of helping.

It has been Colin's lucky day. He has been out on his bean bag under the tree and a couple of engineering students visiting the hospital on a project have seen him, talked to the nursing assistants about his mobility problem (consultation at last!) and promised to build him 'a kind of pram'.

I think everyone concerned has always meant to do something about a chair for Colin, but the problems of everyday life on a busy ward squeeze out such innovations. There are always more pressing needs. Colin cannot make his presence felt, so he gets forgotten.

Whether it is the effects of the extra stimulation, the good weather or an enjoyable tea, the 'babies' are quite different from the last time I saw them, much more animated.

I am sitting on the end of Roddy's bed for some time before I realize that he is raising his head and shoulders off his one pillow and straining to see me. Flat on his back, he can see very little and he is not able to reposition himself.

'He understands a lot of what you say to him,' Jill, the part-timer said. 'I've been asking him if his mother is coming to see him and he almost said "yes". You should see him when she comes – his legs and arms go. He's so excited.'

Sally is luckier. She is mobile enough to change her position. The others lie as they are placed, heads by the walls. The cupboards in between make it hard to see each other or passing staff. Sally has simply done an about-turn and lies with her head at the bottom of the cot and a clear view around the room. She refuses to sleep in any other position.

Immediately after tea the two women start the evening wash-and-change session struggling with unwieldy limbs – 'top and tailing' – only this time, in the cots. The girls are dressed in pretty nightdresses, Roddy and Colin in pyjamas.

Some of the bed linen is wet or soiled and this has to be changed with the patient still in bed, a strenuous job. There is, they have decided rightly, a strange smell from some of the cots and are not sure if it is animal, vegetable or mineral. In the end, they decide it is coming from the patients themselves, rather than the bed linen and put it down to something they ate.

Apart from the distinctive odour of a wet nappy when you lean over a cot occasionally, there was never an unpleasant smell in the room – none of the stale smells associated with this kind of ward. It helped, perhaps, that it was summer, with the windows open. One of the nursing assistants said her husband insists she change her clothes when she gets home at night because they always smell.

'I'm glad we didn't have a handicapped child,' she said. 'I don't think my husband would have been able to cope. I never thought about something going wrong when I was having mine, but I would now if I was pregnant. I would worry all the time. You realize handicapped children can be born to anyone, in any class.'

In fact, they have little to do with parents, because few visit, but they know potted histories of several of the patients. Parents are welcome. One of the girls, whose mother had lost track of her – a nurse shook her head in amazement at this – had turned up on Sunday and everyone hoped she would keep coming.

Despite a life-time of nappies, there is not a bedsore in sight, they point out proudly, as they proceed with bowls of water from cot to cot. The older of the two women, who works full-time, is defensive. 'We do everything that can be done for these kids. There is nothing more a parent could do if they lived at home. In fact they are better looked after here. They get nursing care night and day. If they are ill, day or night, a doctor will be called. You don't get that at home.'

She is right in one way. They are cleaned and fed and their bodies cared for beautifully. Whether they are cared for on an emotional level is open to question – or whether anyone stops to wonder if they have any emotions. All but one of the 'babies' smiled and responded to individual attention. A couple say words or phrases. Everyone who comes into contact with them agrees they are not the vegetables outsiders imagine. But they do need time and patience and familiar faces and voices to get anything out of them.

The nursing officer is aware of their needs. She would like – and is hoping to get – a part-time speech therapist who would spend time with them. She wants to send them to the school at the sister hospital, which takes children to nineteen, if transport could be arranged. There is talk of bringing in volunteers, for a one-to-one stint with each child, once a week. Volunteers are thin on the ground – none of the grass-roots staff I met had ever worked with one – and the hospital did not have a volunteer co-ordinator though they were looking for one.

One nurse pointed out that he and some of his colleagues are against volunteers on principle anyway, because they invalidate their ultimate weapon in any dispute, withdrawal of labour.

It would take a particularly dedicated volunteer to work with these teenagers. There are no instant, easy rewards and they do not have the popular appeal of children. Years of institutional life have taken away much of their individuality – and even the most heavily handicapped person is an individual with a personality as distinct as a thumb-print.

It is easy to point out what could or should be done but, after a couple of hours with the 'babies', you can feel the helplessness a nurse must feel, until she blocks it off. After you have talked to them a little, got a smile, what do you do next? If you could get half-a-dozen words from the most able in as many months, so what? What difference would it make to their lives? Where would you go from there?

One nursing assistant said it used to depress her, but not any more. She has stopped feeling, because it is too painful. 'There is no point. You just do what you can to make them comfortable.'

They have given up on the infant teenagers of Honeysuckle. No one holds out hope now of toilet training, getting them to speak or move. They are doomed to the most dependent kind of babyhood for life.

Need it be like this? With the miracles of physiotherapy, speech therapy, stimulation, affection and attention, they would still have been severely handicapped individuals – but a little less handicapped, a little more individual perhaps, capable of enjoying some part of their restricted lives. They are at the bottom of the pile – not just of this hospital, but everywhere. The ones the stretched resources don't quite reach. The forgotten minority within a minority.

7.45 p.m.

The nursing assistants have had a fifteen-minute tea-break (do staff ever actually eat? I never saw anyone consume anything more filling than a piece of cake – and that was only one nurse!). They have also administered an enema to an old man who is ill in bed, with the help of the trained nurse. Their duties do not end with the 'babies'. If they are not doing something with them, they are expected to lend a hand elsewhere on the ward.

Lastly, they have tucked in their six special charges and got them settled for the night. They lie, firmly positioned between white sheets, none of them showing any inclination to sleep.

It is very quiet, but then this is generally probably the quietest ward in the hospital. There is a small television, but it is rarely turned on because, the nurses say, the 'babies' do not take any notice of it. They wouldn't be able to see it anyway, from a lying position in their cots.

No lights have been turned on, but there is still enough light from outside to see. Colin has his arm under his head and can look around. One of the girls moves her fingers in front of her eyes, watching them with fascination. Sally holds on to her tambourine and makes occasional small noises. There are no playthings in or on the cots. There are no sounds of discontent.

The trained nurse (an SEN), who has been in charge, is going off duty at eight, when night staff come on. She is middle-aged and has worked in the hospital most of her working life. Recently she was on the Children's Ward. 'I didn't want to leave. It broke my heart, but I see now it was right to move me. You get too involved. Over there I saw myself as a mother-figure. Here I am doing some real nursing again.'

Outside working hours, she, like most nurses, has no links with the patients. Nobody takes one or two to their home or out for a day. This particular nurse used to take a group of high-grade boys to her house as part of their training, 'but things started disappearing and turning up on top of their wardrobes. They don't appreciate normal home life.'

Honeysuckle is one of the solid, red-brick, pre-war 'home units'. Upstairs is an adolescent boys' training unit, which runs separately, but with the same nursing officer in charge.

Across the path, there is music coming from the 'rec' – a great blue hut of a building that invites puns. There is a disco in session, the abler young men and women dancing together or standing listening, with their arms around each other. There will be table tennis and card games in a while – but not of course for the Honeysuckle patients. Only one of them – a youngish, physically fit man, goes over there, occasionally, in the evening, and he looks lost.

'It's okay here for the ones who can do a bit for themselves,' one staff member had volunteered, talking about the 'babies'. 'But if I had a child like these little ones, I would want a small home, with plenty of staff. I wouldn't let him come here.'

POPPY WARD – CHILDREN

Poppy Ward is a long, prefabricated building, sectioned off into two main areas by a waist-high 'fence'. The larger section has ten beds with individual lockers and wardrobes beside them. At its furthest end, there is a bathroom and a small laundry room, with automatic machine and dryer, where the ward's washing is done.

In the centre, where it meets the play area, is the nurses' office and a small dining section, with two tables and a collection of chairs. There is a tiny kitchen, where food brought from the staff dining-room is heated and served. On the other side of the barricade, with a gate which is bolted, is the play area, with a television, plenty of toys, a trampoline and a big day mattress on the floor. At the end of this are four toilets and four washbasins. There are posters on the walls, a carpet in the play area, which has just been re-decorated. It is bright and cheerful. Nobody pretends it is ideal – it was intended only as an interim ward – but it is adequate, give or take a few problems, such as the need for a second bath which they have been promised.

There were no children at the hospital until three years ago – other hospitals in the group had taken them. The nursing officer in charge had never been responsible for mentally handicapped children before and was worried about how they should be cared for. 'Then I decided to treat them like normal children. They are children first, after all.'

She is still intensely aware, though, of the emotional issues surrounding the whole idea of children in hospitals. She had just read Maureen Oswin's damning account *Children Living in Long Stay Hospitals* and been very affected by it.

'Do you know she mentions cases of children getting only five minutes' mothering in a day. No touching or cuddling at all. I rushed over to the ward to tell them this and when I got here, there were two nurses cuddling two children on their laps. It made me feel a bit better.'

The hospital is not geared to children. Some people think it is the last place they should be, with locked wards and an interim secure unit opening soon. But in one way, being a minority group is an advantage. The children have a novelty value they would not achieve in a hospital where there were masses of them. Staff from other wards tend to drop in. The more able patients do the same. The nurses, mostly mothers themselves, get quite emotional over them.

Whether all this makes the children's lives any better is hard to say. What everyone agrees they need is more staff, and I don't think any clever juggling of people or rearranging of duties can get away from it here. It is an exhausting ward to work on, particularly at weekends and during school holidays.

'On Honeysuckle they don't run away or go outside and eat leaves off the trees,' one nurse said. 'You can sit down and have a cup of tea. Here you are on duty every minute. You never stop.'

8.30 a.m.

Breakfast is half-way through on Poppy. Four of the nine children living there at the moment (the population fluctuates, because a few children come in on a short-stay basis) are seated around two tables, eating sausages, tomatoes and fried bread out of dishes, with varying degrees of competence. One of them, a teenage girl, is in her wheelchair. Two physically handicapped children are being fed, in low chairs, and two more are waiting their turn in the play area. The feeding chairs look fairly inappropriate and women doing the feeding have to get down on one knee to get at the children.

Running hither and thither, stark naked – the others are in nightclothes – is an exceptionally good-looking boy of around nine. This is Guy. He is autistic and, without doubt, the child who gives the staff the most headaches. I never once saw him fully dressed. Everything put on him is immediately removed, unless the staff can find some clever way of stopping him stripping.

The night-nurse buttons his pyjamas down the back, ensuring a minimum of covering. When he wakes in the early hours of the morning and disturbs the other children by running around or getting into their beds, she takes him down to the play area. Often, she says, she rocks him to sleep again in her arms, lays him down wherever he happens to be and covers him with a blanket.

She changes nappies and gets the children up whenever they wake, from around 5 a.m. onwards. Later sleepers are got up at 6.45 a.m. to be ready for the day staff coming on at 8 a.m. to start breakfast.

There are four nurses on this morning – one young girl 'borrowed' regularly from a workshop, for a hectic hour, two mature women 'regulars' and a young, trendy male charge nurse, who has been there only a couple of months. It seems a reasonable staff ratio, but he says he needs five staff at busy times like breakfast. He never, of course, gets them. Nor does he hold out hope of getting the other facility he would most like – a mini-bus to take the children out which he could drive himself, instead of waiting for hospital transport. 'Union problems' are blamed for preventing this.

Breakfast is reasonably uneventful. Paul, a tall thirteen-year-old, partially sighted West Indian boy, gets upset about something and lashes out alarmingly. One of the women wraps her arms around him and calms him down. 'He doesn't do this often, but he can land a punch. He's lovely most of the time, aren't you Paul?' Paul responds with a smile.

One little girl who can walk, but is fed with the physically handicapped group, is tied in a chair to be given her breakfast. She rocks and bangs about continually and half the food ends up on her face and clothes. This is Susan, not a pretty child, but a great giggler, very responsive and plainly everybody's favourite. Outsiders and ward staff alike tickle her and tease and play with her. She not only gets her share of mothering, but a bit of everyone else's as well.

8.40 a.m.

The bathing starts. Each child is bathed every morning and often has his hair washed, too. As there is only bath in a small bathroom and they go in one at a time, with fresh water for each (not so usual as it might sound), it is squashed and frantic at the bottom end of the dormitory. One child is left shivering and naked waiting to go in next, another is pushed out and left shivering even more until someone can get round to washing and dressing her. The heating is on and the staff are sweating, but sitting in a wheelchair wet is still pretty goose-pimpling. To be fair, they are not left for long. Everything is done at a pace, a bath taking around three minutes, because the bus to take them to another hospital school five miles away arrives around 9.15 a.m. They commandeer four of the nearest beds, covered with rubber sheeting and use these for drying and dressing the children. At first two dress and two bath. When the bathing is over, the other two join in the dressing. Instead of towelling nappies each child wears disposable nappy pads – two or three – covered by tie plastic pants. ('These nappies are useless. You have to keep changing them every five minutes and they are uncomfortable. I wouldn't use them,' one nursing assistant with young children of her own, informed me on another shift.)

The clothes are of good quality, none of the rag-bag hospital look the 'babies' on the other ward have. Some wards, and this is one of them, have a £30 clothing allowance for each resident, and staff go out and buy individual items. Pathetic though the sum is, it seems to work, supplemented by hospital issue for basics. Each child has his or her own clothes washed and ironed on the ward – the care staff do that too – so they do not get lost or damaged in a big central laundry. The parents who see their children regularly do, of course, supply some clothing, but this accounts for only about half the number.

Finance is confusing. Each long-term child gets pocket money, some of which is banked and used for outings and holidays – the annual trip to Colwyn Bay – and special clothes for such events. The rest of the pocket money is spent for them on sweets and treats from the hospital shop. Nurses rarely handle money and have a shopping card for each child.

One of the full-time nursing assistants, Janet, goes to school with the children and helps out there during the day with the Poppy Ward children. It is a good idea, on paper, giving a sense of continuity to the children. The school is modern and grand, with specialists like hospital physiotherapists, to spare. In theory, ward nurses should know what each child is doing there and continue it on the ward.

In fact, there is little time to do anything but see to bodily needs on the ward and, according to another nurse who used to do the hospital-school trip, ward staff are resented and not made good use of at the school. One nurse, given the opportunity, would change the system and keep the children on the ward all day, employing more staff to work with them on stimulation programmes and having a physio and speech therapist come in.

'We could do so much more here if we had enough help and it would not be so disruptive as taking them out to school.'

Janet, a mother of teenagers, who gave up an office job that paid twice her present salary 'because this was something I always wanted to do', is plainly suited to the job. She is a naturally affectionate woman, who touches and cuddles children automatically. There is little scope for it, though. There is not, she admits, as much child-care as she wanted and expected in the job.

'I just wish there was more time to play with them,' she said. It seems a sad waste of a talent that is rarer than it should be in this line of work.

By 9.15 a.m., when I left, all but the last two children were dressed, combed and tidied. The nurses, from so much tugging and pushing and manipulating of arms and legs, looked worn out. Guy was half-way through undressing yet again.

Tuesday 5 p.m. – Bank Holiday week

A sweltering hot day and it still has not cooled down comfortably. Most of the children are in the play area, sitting listlessly or wandering about, agitated. Several are sunburnt – at least one girl has been blistered – but that was from yesterday, another scorcher. Some are crying. All are unhappy.

There is a playground at the back with swings and big toys and they have all been out a lot over the weekend. Today, they have been kept inside.

Paul, though, is outside the main double doors in just his plastic pants, laughing as he moves his hand between his eyes and the sun; wandering off a few yards to pull leaves off a tree and chew them experimentally.

'It doesn't seem to do him any harm,' one of the nurses said. The youngest child on the ward – a frail, physically handicapped six-year-old, is lying in her cot, the only bed with sides. The rest are ordinary divans with attractive, bright bedspreads. There are some elaborate toys hanging on the cot – mobiles, musical movement toys – and a three-dimensional poster of kittens above her bed. She takes little notice of anything, or anyone. Her mother has not visited her for a long time.

Angela, too, is in the dormitory area. She lies immobile on a bed on her back, with only the ceiling to look at; a long thin, delicate-boned girl of thirteen. A contender to join the 'babies' of Honeysuckle later, I would imagine, with her spastic limbs and total dependency. She is the sort of child who gets ignored because she never asks for attention. At first, she looks totally unresponsive, immersed in her own world, but when I lean over to look directly at her, she smiles and watches with interest. A hanging cot toy with bells has fallen off the smaller girl's bed. There is no place to hang it within view of Angela, so I try putting it in her hand. She clutches it, waves it around, big brown eyes growing wider with excitement, while I wonder nervously if she might hurt herself, if that is the reason she did not already have a toy. She doesn't seem to be. When, half-an-hour later, she is transferred to one of those low chairs for feeding, she is still holding it, still animated.

Janet, who has been on duty since 8 a.m., has no time for worrying about handing out toys or seeing to plaintive moans. The food has just been delivered and she has to see to doling it out and feeding. She keeps on the move between the kitchen and the office, where, with the help of another nurse, she is sorting out drugs. Several of the children need drugs to control epilepsy. Angela has something for muscle spasm and there are always odds and ends like laxatives for those who need them. Mundane details like this are filled in daily in a record book.

Because of holiday leave, Janet has virtually been on her own on the ward all day, with people 'popping over for an hour or so from other wards' to help out. Just before tea, at 5.30 p.m., an evening part-timer arrives. The nurse who helped with the drugs, now distributed, has left.

Together in the kitchen, they put out portions of potato and fish-fingers (or is it rissoles? it's hard to tell) with something that looks like chicken soup poured over it. When they turn their backs, one of the taller boys, Gerry, leans across the half-partition, gets hold of a ladle and ladles soup all over the place.

A pretty little girl, just tall enough to bang her head on the top of the partition, does so, and there is some alarm. She has had three stitches in her forehead already today – the result of falling forward with a fit.

There are four self-feeders today. One boy is a new face to me – a 'short stay', with an alarming habit of turning blue. None of the nurses seems sure what causes it, but there are some confused explanations.

I am given Angela to feed, because she is the easiest, and the part-timer feeds the multiply handicapped six-year-old, who in fact eats next to nothing. The nurse gets cramp from her crouching position for her efforts.

Angela eats all the mushy mixture very slowly. 'She is a real little lady, only sips her drinks and takes tiny mouthfuls,' Janet says, giving her a squeeze in passing. Faced with treacle tart for afters, though, she spits it out in a very unladylike manner. 'Don't worry, just leave it,' I am told. 'If they don't eat, we can't force them.'

The other two are working their way through feeding at a rapid rate. The four at the table have more food on themselves, the floor and the chairs than in their mouths. They are supposed to be able to feed themselves, but a couple of them, at least, really cannot manage the complicated manoeuvre of loading a spoon and getting it, still full, to their mouths.

The short-stay boy is lucky if he gets half the meal and the two women are far too involved with feeding the physically handicapped ones to help him. Paul manages only by dispensing with his cutlery and picking it up with his hands. One of the women, in passing, firmly puts a spoon back in his hand. Teaching social skills, or trying to implement what they may have picked up at school, is impossible. Are there usually more staff, I wonder? 'No,' they say. Often there are just two of them, sometimes there are three.

No bibs or protective garments of any kind are worn – perhaps it is considered an assault on the dignity of older children. There are no tissues or kitchen rolls – anything that might be used to wipe and throw away. Not for the first time, I wonder why such modern conveniences are non-existent in all the residential establishments. Nobody in their right mind feeds a baby or a handicapped child at home without some convenient 'wipe' at hand. How would you like to eat your dinner with your whole face and half your body covered in gravy and mash? Disposable bibs and tissues are available to wards for the asking, senior hospital staff insist. But then why are they not asked for? All clothing is changed daily – twice a day if you count nightclothes. They have to be. Janet says: 'It's the mess that gets you down. The place is in a continual mess.'

Afterwards there is a drink, orange squash. All the children are desperately thirsty. Janet says they have been drinking all day and they are almost out of squash. Most of them, I'm sure, would quite happily drink tap water rather than nothing. Those who can indicate they want more, get more. Those who cannot ask, like Angela, get one cup. One boy, Simon, who is spastic, is so excited, he cannot, for a while, get his teeth round the spouted cup which is being held for him. He makes several involuntary lunges before he and the cup get together.

He is a fairly difficult child, Simon, simply because he loves attention and will often cry continually until he is taken out of his chair or until someone sits beside him and talks exclusively to him. He sees his parents and goes home for visits and is, unlike the children who know nothing else, intensely aware of the difference between being one of a family and one of a large group.

He does get some of the attention he demands, more than most. During the evening Janet had him on her lap for two sessions. Once when she was having a cup of tea before going off duty, illustrating the fact that you never get away from the job on Poppy. Neither is it possible to apportion attention equally. Inevitably the most demanding get most.

A quick sort-out of individuals before bath-time: two children who can go to the toilet with a bit of help are taken down to the washroom at the play area end. An under-used place this, because most of them are in nappies and totally dependent. One boy is hot and agitated and has not eaten anything. He may be sickening for something and a report has to be made.

A cleaner comes in to mop out the dining area – the only job the nurses don't do – and the children are moved on to beds or into the play area, while the two women get ready to 'top and tail' them for the night. This is done on two beds at the lower end of the dormitory, with just two bowls of water on a trolley and no individual cloths. Half-way through, there is screaming and shouting from the far end of the ward and Janet remembers she left Nicholas on the toilet. 'He's so quiet you forget about him.'

Nicholas, brought down for washing, has a face like thunder. Suddenly, sitting on the bed, he begins to bang his fist against his head and face. Janet tries to stop him, tries to soothe him, then, helplessly, lets him continue. She has never seen him behave like this. There is no explanation. The cleaner joins in. She thinks the boy who is in for a short stay may have bitten him. She has just spotted him trying to do it to another child up that end. He is taken down to where an eye can be kept on him. Nicholas calms down, though he looks gravely affronted. He is the oldest in the ward, rarely visited, 'but his father's secretary rings up to ask how he is'. At nearly nineteen, he is old for the ward. 'I think they worry about the homosexuality on the men's wards. He is not able to defend himself. He would be very vulnerable,' a nurse told me.

A 'high-grade' teenage girl who lives in a detached house in the grounds, part of a group training to live in the community, comes in to chat. She plays with Susan who is being washed and changed. She has been out shopping and shows us her dress material. 'I don't tell people where I come from,' she says. 'They think it's a mad house.' 'She is only here,' one of the staff tells me, 'because nobody seemed to know quite where to put her.' Certainly she mixes more easily with staff than residents.

Another visitor is a middle-aged nurse from the next ward. She wants to know if Guy is coming back tonight. If so, they will have to close all the windows, however the temperature soars. Had he been there over the stifling weekend, doors and windows would have had to be locked to stop him getting out and running away. Fortunately his parents took him home, but his mother had rung to say she didn't think she could cope and might have to bring him back. Nobody seemed sure if he was coming, but at this late stage it was thought improbable. 'He doesn't belong in this ward,' somebody says. 'We haven't the facilities to help him and the other children suffer because of him.' Rumour has it a place is being sought for him in a boarding school, but there is a desperate shortage of places for the 'Guys' of the world.

7.45 p.m.

All the children are in nightclothes and night nappies. Most are in their beds, Susan banging her head on the headboard, but it is padded specifically because of this. She doesn't have visitors. She was a normal baby, until she was battered by her parents.

The little girl with stitches is left in the play area because she is known not to settle in bed until later. She sits in a chair, holding a soft toy, sucking her thumb. The television, protected by a sort of fence, has not been on. 'It is on sometimes, but they never watch it,' one nurse said. 'They don't play either, none of them, despite all the toys. You have to be on your own with one of them and try really hard before they will.'

One-to-one in any residential situation is a pipe-dream, but the nursing officer, like all good people, has a dream. She has twenty hours of 'person time' to play around with it, it seems, and she hopes to get two play leaders for ten hours at weekends, 'purely to come in and play with the children'.

Janet, to whom I mentioned this, would understandably prefer to spend ten hours playing with the children herself and let someone else do ten hours of donkey-work.

Community Homes

'Small is beautiful' and 'Community' is trendy. So there is a tendency to prefix everything smaller than a hospital with the word community. It can get confusing.

Basically a community home, to state the obvious, should be in the community, so that residents live in close proximity to shops, transport, neighbours and other delights and irritations of normal life. It is the natural backlash to all the decades of isolated institutions.

It should be homely, small and as much like a family home in day-to-day running as possible. Those criteria satisfied, a community home is in the eye of the beholder. Location, architecture, staffing and choice of residents can vary tremendously.

Such homes have been set up by Local Authorities and by voluntary organizations. Others, like Oakengates and Bridge House, are 'satellite' homes to a mental handicap hospital. They are administered by the hospital group, serviced by the hospital, but function with a degree of autonomy – although a nurse at one of them pointed out: 'We have to accept that we cannot do just what we fancy here. We are always bound by the rules and regulations of the hospital.'

Both homes have six beds for children under sixteen, but Bridge House had an empty bed and some uncertainty about its future. There has been talk of its being used for short-stay. It would be ideal, but, on the other hand, it seems a pity to deprive a further group of long-stay children of the only chance they will have of a home life.

Both places serve up as many home comforts as you are likely to find in residential care. For the children they cater for – medium dependency in Oakengates, fairly self-sufficient in Bridge House – they are among the better solutions.

Oakengates is a sturdy, detached, family house with a big garden, at the edge of a built-up area and within walking distance of the hospital. Bridge House was two three-bedroomed police houses with a small surburban station between. As the home is five miles away from the hospital, except for specialists who visit, the children themselves have little contact with that institution.

They are, with the exception of the newest arrival, easy, sociable teenagers. You could, you feel, put them down anywhere and they would live happily. But, as Mr J, the charge nurse, pointed out, I was seeing them after three years there – years of homely living and incidental training. When they arrived, hand-picked as the most likely to succeed in this experimental attempt at normalization, they were 'institutionalized, unsociable and lacking initiative or individuality'.

The Oakengates children are noticeably more handicapped. A nursing assistant with no previous experience who had just started work there when the first batch arrived, remembers expecting a bunch of sweet, helpless little souls – and being shocked by the reality. 'They were little animals.' They have all – again with the exception of one – responded to individual attention and improved greatly.

It is some measure of the pull of the place that the lady who was initially shocked is still there. 'You get involved with the children,' she said. 'They say you shouldn't, but I don't think you would do this job otherwise. You are the only family they know. They turn to you for love and comfort.'

Staff do seem to last in the homes. That is one of the strengths. Untrained staff for the most part – local women who work full or part-time to fit in with family commitments. One young woman took maternity leave when her second child was born and went back to a shift adapted to suit her, starting at 5 p.m.

Incidentally it allows her to work, at some stage, with everyone and gives her a unique view of where continuity and consistency of training and handling break down, which she can point out at staff meetings.

In the other home, a part-timer whose children are now able to look after themselves for a while, has become a full-timer. Arrangements are fluid and easy-going. It helps to attract the sort of person needed – jacks of all trades and masters of quite a few.

Everyone who works in the homes 'mucks in'. Nursing assistants look after the children, take them out, cook meals, change nappies if needed, sweep floors, do the washing. There are domestics, but they do more than pushing a vacuum cleaner around. The situation in practice is something like a housewife with a mother's help. The demarcation line is hazy.

At Oakengates, one of the domestics changed and washed the only child in nappies when care staff were busy. At Bridge House after she had finished her work, the cleaner sat watching television with one of the girls on her lap.

Each home has a male charge nurse – a bachelor in one, a young married man in the other – and a trained deputy, both female. The two men are different in temperament and their attitude to the job, but both talk of similar problems, experienced in a situation very different from the hospital wards where they worked previously.

They had to get used to being, virtually, at home all day – the kind of isolation women are traditionally more used to coping with. They have had to adapt to working very closely in an informal set-up with untrained staff – and all female at that.

Mr J at Bridge House was particularly aware of the isolation, being furthest from the hospital. 'You miss the male companionship, meeting your mates for a drink at lunch-time. A place like this was the pipe-dream of every nurse, when there were four of us on a ward with eighty patients. Imagine what you could do with just half-a-dozen kids. It is perfect for the kids – but it can create problems for those in charge.'

Communication problems can crop up. One of the men explained: 'I'd been used to working with other trained nurses and talking in medical terminology. I have to remember to simplify everything. At first I found that if I gave some instructions and they were not working, nobody would come and tell me. They would just carry on regardless, unquestioning, while everyone got more and more frustrated.'

Both men discovered that they had to emphasize the time it might take for a child to master a particular skill, that results would not happen overnight – something inexperienced staff have to find out the hard way.

'I don't think the people up at the hospital take us seriously if we mention managerial problems because this is so small-scale,' one of them said. 'But they exist. Working as close as this to people, you have to tread a very fine line to get the balance right.'

Some of the nursing assistants are acutely conscious of their lack of knowledge and would like the chance to learn – in the right way. One of them said: 'I wish sometimes I knew how to teach the children, how to play with them constructively. I just use my head and the experience I've gained with my own children. I'd like to learn a lot more about these children and how to help them. It has to be the right teacher, though, someone who doesn't talk over your head.'

Some of the women had done a short in-service training. One of them felt it did not apply to the mildly handicapped children in her care. Another had been told she didn't need to do a course as she had taken one in her previous hospital job. 'Not that there was much similarity. It was all about dealing with sick people and laying out the dead.' Senior staff insist that a course is offered to everyone eventually and in turn. They cannot all be fitted in at once.

Both homes have basic practical ties with the hospital. Their larder supplies and household items come from there. Meals are normally cooked on the spot but, if there are staff shortages or any other drama, they can be sent over from the hospital kitchens.

They have their share of hospital transport. The Bridge House children had used the mini-bus for outings during the summer holiday. The Oakengates residents are taken for a drive every Sunday, rain or shine. Both homes take part in hospital special days and holidays, as well as any additional ones staff like to organize and fund-raise for.

A nursing officer is in daily contact. A consultant psychiatrist calls as a routine. A psychologist is available to assess individual children and work out programmes for the staff to use. And indeed both homes currently have a problem child, straining the collective ingenuity.

Oakengates children go to school at the hospital. Bridge House residents to the local special school. There are similarities, but there are differences, too. Bridge House *has* to involve itself with the community because the hospital is too far away to lean on, so it is perhaps the truest to its name.

I have, incidentally, called one charge nurse by his Christian name and the other by his surname, because this happens to be the way they style themselves to staff, children and visitors.

OAKENGATES

Monday 4.30 p.m.

The children have been home for a hour, escorted by one of the staff. They are out in the garden doing their own thing. They do not play together, though there is a swing, a sand pit and plenty of large toys. Malcolm is on the swing. Sandy hovers between house and garden, clutching a doll and keeping an eye on the adults. Nancy rocks in a garden chair not meant for rocking. Brenda is not in sight or too silent to be noticed. Ronnie pursues his obsession with tractors, gazing at one working in the next field. James runs hither and thither, lies on the ground, shouts.

James is the problem. A slender, good-looking boy of eleven, he is causing more worry than the other five put together. He arrived from the hospital eighteen months ago – a mistake, many of the staff now feel. He soon became aggressive, attacking staff and children and hitting his own face 'until he looked like he'd gone ten rounds with Muhammad Ali'.

The staff were convinced there was a simple, logical, physical explanation – toothache or headache, even a brain tumour. The hospital support services were called in. No physical cause could be found. It is not that he does not feel pain – he will cry if he falls over and hurts himself or if he is smacked.

'We finally had to accept that he was hurting himself – and to a lesser extent other people – for attention.' Hazel, a nursing assistant, said. 'I couldn't believe it at first, but I do now. He is very masochistic, and he enjoys seeing other children suffer, too. When he gets his own way, he has this gloating little smile on his face. I think if he cannot be helped, James will grow up to be a very dangerous man.'

It is hard to see him like that now, though. He just looks a confused, unhappy little boy. He goes from room to room – the children have the run of the house – lying on the floor sometimes, throwing a ball to the charge nurse after some encouragement.

Both his arms are in restraining splints, held on by velcro. Not uncomfortable and he could remove them himself, but he wants them there. They were put on originally to stop him hitting his face. Now the problem is to get him to manage without them before they become a fixture. Immediately one is removed, he smashes his fist against his chin and whimpers until the restraint is replaced.

A psychologist from the hospital has worked out a programme for James mainly to curtail his aggression, now directed almost entirely inwards, but also to get him toilet trained and able to wash and feed himself more capably.

The staff, though, sound defeated about him. They hold out little hope of success. There is a feeling that they may have to ask to have him sent back to the hospital, but this will rest on the final decision of the hospital consultant.

'As a result of James's problems the other children are becoming disturbed because we cannot give them their share of attention,' Gary points out. 'We've started getting soiled pants and temper tantrums – two sure ways for them to get attention, too.'

5.30 p.m.

The other children *look* fairly happy. They come in to sit round a table in the small dining-room which adjoins a large kitchen. It is unpretentious, clean, very ordinary. Vinyl on the floor, a plastic table-cloth. They had tea and cake when they came in from school. Now they get a plate heaped with fish fingers, chips and peas.

Iris, a new nursing assistant who used to work at the hospital, has cooked it. There is no set menu, because they cannot rely on getting exactly what they order from the hospital stores. Meals are prepared from what turns up. If anything is missing, there is a small shopping centre within walking distance. Someone will go round and take one or two of the children for a treat. The children could not go alone.

The staff do not have a meal with them but Hazel, who is on duty until nine o'clock and Gary who is on till eight, with Iris, supervise. All the children can cope with knives and forks, except James who has been persuaded to hold a knife but not yet to use it. They have learned this skill at Oakengates, along with toilet training. In the hospital there was no one with the time to try and teach them.

Fourteen-year-old Sandy, painfully thin, is the only problem eater. She simply doesn't, despite drugs to give her an appetite. When she first came she was on a special diet, because it was thought that her system could not take ordinary food. Home for Christmas with one of the staff, she tested the seasonal goodies, uninvited – and suffered no ill effects. Gradually everyday items were introduced to her diet and she is none the worse for it, except that she is still a small eater. The staff now insist her digestive problems were psychological all along. She is even credited with being able to control her bowels at will, just to annoy.

If you can talk of success and failure in this setting, Sandy, amiable and sociable though she is, is a failure. She understands a lot, but she will never, it now seems, be able to look after herself in the simplest fashion. When she reaches sixteen, instead of transferring to a hostel, which was the aim for all six children, she will probably go back to a hospital ward.

You have to be realistic, Gary points out. Out of the six, he estimates two will go to hostels, two back to hospital and the fate of the remaining pair is still in the balance. When Sandy was taken home for Christmas by Phyl, one of the domestics, she fitted in happily and behaved beautifully. She responds to a real family, everyone agrees, but what family would foster a severely retarded, physically unattractive fourteen-year-old?

Malcolm is one of the lucky ones, who is likely to go on to a hostel. He is a plump, normal-looking boy of eleven – very pernickety, determined that everything in the house is in its rightful place. He eats every scrap of his meal, in strict order, vegetables first, then potatoes, then fish. He will never accept a second portion. Malcolm can dress and undress, wash and go the toilet, without reminders or supervision. He does little jobs like putting out the cutlery or tidying up. He is the most emotionally normal of the children. The biggest problem is that he cannot speak.

They are working on it at Oakengates. Before he is allowed to go after meals, Gary makes him say 'Please may I leave the table'. It sounds like gibberish, but it is a consistent attempt at speech and he is making the effort. They are hoping to get a speech therapist from the hospital to visit him.

There is trifle for dessert. Nancy eats a bit, then plays with it with her spoon, glancing from beneath long, curly eyelashes, to gauge the effect she is making. She is, at ten, the youngest, and another child with high hopes of a hostel place. She is also, the staff say, bright enough to play to the gallery, to manipulate people and to 'try it on' with any newcomer.

'Nancy knows how to twist people round her little finger,' Hazel said, 'but she can really try your patience. I hate the attitude of "I'll tell Daddy" and I would never say it at home or here, but to be honest she behaves better and jumps to it quicker for a man. Gary can handle her better than any of us. It is essential to have a man in this set-up. I think myself we could do with a couple more.'

On a previous visit at lunch-time, Nancy had misbehaved and Gary had made her stand outside the door, watching the others eat. Then she came in to have her lunch alone. Hospital rules and the Mental Health Act do not officially permit physical punishment, 'but we do give them a smack occasionally, exactly as you would a normal child,' he said. 'It would be dishonest to say otherwise.' They also work to the behaviour modification principle of rewarding good behaviour and ignoring the bad – 'harder to do but the effect is longer-lasting'.

None of the staff had meals with the children while I was there – there was little room to spare at the table – although they say they do sit down and have a drink with them. They were either serving food, in the kitchen or supervising. It tends to detract a little from the 'happy family around the table' idea, but is, perhaps, what happens in a lot of hectic households with real, large families.

Staff levels are luxurious by hospital standards, with one charge nurse, one senior enrolled nurse, five nursing assistants, and two domestics, on the payroll. But Gary thinks they need yet more staff. 'You have to think of holidays. For forty-four weeks of the year, we are one person short due to holiday leave – and what about all the time lost through illness?'

There have been times when just one person is left in charge, not easy while they have a child as difficult as James. If a problem arises at any hour of the day or night and there is nobody qualified to deal with it, help can be summoned from the hospital by phone or Gary, who lives nearby, sent for. A local GP is called in the normal way to treat the children – Nancy recently had to be rushed to the nearest general hospital for an operation – and specialist services like dentistry and chiropody are available at the hospital.

Tea over, the children go back into the garden or to the playroom – an indoor room with plenty of toys and birds in a cage. The birds are soon to go – they have been blamed for causing an outbreak of boils.

The children revert to their previous isolated occupations, except for Nancy who stays indoors in the playroom. The staff supervise rather than join in or instigate games, except for Gary attempting to throw a ball to James, which amuses the child for a few minutes.

Hazel sweeps up outside. A part-time domestic help is dealing with indoor cleaning. There is a lot of discussion over who broke a branch off the plum tree. No culprit is found, though Malcolm is suspected. Some of the enterprising ladies have collected plums and made pies, picked blackberries growing in the hedge for similar culinary purposes.

Hazel says she treats the children as if they were, simply, younger, and finds they have a lot in common with her four-year-old. There is some discussion about Nancy and why she wrecked the classroom on her first day back at school, and about the mysterious working of Sandy's bowels. Very mundane stuff.

The staff obviously know and like the children, warts and all, without being sentimental. 'I gave myself three months when I first came,' said Hazel. 'If I started feeling sorry for them, I decided I would leave. You can't be any help to them if you are thinking of them as poor little things.'

Getting to know thirty patients in a hospital ward as well as this would be impossible. There children were a case, a face in the crowd, looked after by a stream of efficient but over-stretched people who probably never got close enough to be irritated by their annoying little habits or moved by their emotions. ('The first time I saw

Malcolm cry, I cried, too,' said one nurse. 'He was so genuinely upset, so normal.')

Only one child, Brenda, the most withdrawn, has regular visits from her mother. The staff at Oakengates and the other children are their family. I cannot see that staff being involved to this extent can be other than a plus, but it makes it even more important to get the right staff and give them the proper skills.

7.10 p.m.

Gary is upstairs in the small cluttered room that serves as an office, filling in the official report for the day, stating that all is well at the time of writing. James's restraints are mentioned, but no other dramas make the news tonight. The night nurse will add her remarks in the mornings.

There is only one person (untrained) on each night and she has to get the children who need it out of bed for toileting. There has been trouble recently because two night nurses manage to produce dry children in the morning and the third, wet children. Another close-range management problem.

8 p.m.

Jill, the night nurse, and Hazel are supervising changing and washing upstairs. In their own room, with a lot of urging from Hazel, the three girls change into night-dresses, dressing-gowns and slippers. The boys do the same next door, with some loud verbal encouragement from Jill.

The two rooms are adequately sized, with carpets, modern beds and a wardrobe/chest unit by each. Each child has his or her own clothes, all reasonably attractive and plentiful. It turns out that Phyl is a dab hand at making and adapting clothes and staff and friends regularly bring in second-hand items.

The Home does a little independent fund-raising, quite apart from anything the League of Friends at the hospital might contribute. A local club donated, to them recently, £200 raised in an evening, and Gary is thinking of approaching local firms which might make donations or take an interest in an individual child. A letter to a tractor manufacturer brought a big poster (now on the wall in the boys' room) and some literature, to fire Ronnie's obsession with tractors.

Dressed for bed, the children wash, one by one, in the bathroom, with varying degrees of assistance.

Downstairs in the dining-room there is a milky drink and biscuits for the children. Then everyone moves to the sitting-room. 'I like to put them in here for half-an-hour or so to quieten them down before bed,' Jill explains. If anything, they look livelier. Ronnie keeps trying to drag me into the garden to look for tractors. Nancy rocks violently in a chair in which she has been forbidden to rock. There are sharp words from Jill. The girl runs out and is retrieved and brought back in tears, to sit sullenly on a settee, still rocking.

The television is on, as it has been most of the evening but, then as now, none of the children watches it. Their attention spans are short. They do watch 'Top of the Pops', though, and Ronnie, to everyone's amusement, has taken to making appreciative noises about the dancers. One of the staff remarked, half-seriously, that it could be more troublesome than his interest in tractors, if it became an obsession.

8.30 p.m.

Hazel, who has collected all the day's clothing and put it in the automatic washing-machine, is in the sitting-room, repairing a pair of trousers. Jill has taken the children up to bed. Three of them have drugs, given out by Gary before he went off, for epilepsy and, in James's case, to quieten him down.

'I didn't believe in drugs for children,' Hazel said, 'until I saw one of them having fits when we cut down the dose.'

Once in bed, they usually go to sleep quickly, though James may wake in the night. Sometimes Jill sits on Nancy's bed until she drops off, because she is the most likely to come back downstairs.

It is the first of Jill's three nights on, followed by three off. She will see to any night toileting that needs doing and get them up in the morning, do the washing and drying, maybe do a bit of ironing and make a pie for tomorrow's lunch. 'It's a bit like having a second home,' she said wryly.

Wednesday 6.40 a.m.

The children, still in nightclothes and dressing-gowns, are having their breakfast – corn-flakes, bacon and beans, with tea, prepared by Jill. It is an earlier than normal start because the assistant who comes in from 7 to 11 a.m. daily is away and Jill has to cope single-handed.

On a normal school day they would have been called at seven o'clock. Today it was 6.20, starting with the boys – getting them up, to the toilet and to wash their hands one by one. Then, after she had made the beds, on to the girls' rooms and the process repeated.

Jill had prepared breakfast before calling them, so they could come straight down to find the corn-flakes on the table.

7.30 a.m.

Jill has finished the washing-up and is having a cup of tea and a cigarette at the kitchen table, while she fills in the 'communication' book. This is a ledger in which staff write casual notes of the night's or day's happenings for the next person on duty: essential with several people working there.

The book covers anything, from who has been to the toilet to reminders to order kitchen supplies. Today, she asks for more washing powder. There is an exercise book entirely devoted to James – remarks about his behaviour for the next person to take over.

The children are dotted about all over the place. Malcolm has been sent upstairs to get his clothes on – the only one who can manage this feat alone. Nancy is in the sitting-room, where the record player is on full-blast. When the record ends she comes in and asks for another.

James is in the hall, lying on the floor, screaming from time to time. There are two large bruises on his chin. Jill thinks he did one this morning, when his splints were off for him to eat breakfast. Sometimes one will fall off in bed at night and he will wake up screaming.

Ronnie is upstairs on the toilet. Sandy and Brenda are in the two downstairs toilets. 'I leave them there until they do something,' Jill said. What if they don't need to? 'They will – it's a regular morning routine.' Two of the three reappear within ten minutes, but nearly an hour later someone has to go to fetch Brenda.

Phyl, the domestic who works until lunch-time, has arrived just after 7.30. Her shift starts at eight, but she is always early and does more helping with the children – tying Malcolm's shoe-laces, finding the forgotten Brenda and helping her dress – until they have gone to school.

Gary arrives early, too, and makes tea. There is some discussion on Sandy, the non-eater, demolishing two helpings of curry the previous night. Sandy, who has joined the adults around the table, clutching yet another doll, looks pleased with herself. Phyl says that if she didn't have to go to work, she would foster Sandy, rather than have to see her go back to hospital.

When Jill goes off duty, Malcolm fetches her coat, helps her on with it, walks her to the door and kisses her. Iris, the second member of the care staff on duty, has arrived by then – and the children are rounded up for dressing and washing upstairs, in the crowded bathroom (two wash-basins, one bath, own toothbrushes and face cloths) in that order.

It is an on-going social training programme of the kind not possible in hospital. Gary stands behind Ronnie, holding his hands in the water, helping him lather them and rub them over his face. A half-hearted second splash of the soapy water serves as rinsing and Ronnie is left to dry a face still covered in rich lather. The peculiar refusal in Homes and hospitals to rinse off soap extends to here. Next, Ronnie reluctantly cleans his teeth, with a hand firmly over his.

The process is repeated with the other children, after they are helped to dress by Iris. She takes James for washing, growing irritated with him as he tries to sit on the floor and refuses to co-operate in any way. He seems to inspire an unreasonable amount of annoyance in otherwise patient people.

His splints, of course, are off. He whimpers continually and thrusts his arms at the adults for help. The previous day there was a case conference on him, with everyone called in to discuss his problems and offer suggestions – psychiatrist, psychologist, teacher, social worker, nursing officer and charge nurse.

The sum of their combined experience has produced a new behaviour modification programme carefully and simply written out in longhand for all the Oakengates staff to understand and a new solution to the splint problem.

James is to have plaster of paris on both arms, chipped off so gradually over several weeks that he will not notice the difference. Eventually, he will be left with two bracelet-width pieces around his wrists, which should give him the psychological security he seems to crave.

I make a mental note to check up on James and this unlikely solution in six months. 'You never really know what will work,' Gary admits. 'You have to give it a try.' Defeatist that I am, I would be inclined to leave the boy wearing these two comfortable, removable, elbow-high appliances which look like strips of boned corset for as long as he needs them. They serve the purpose of preventing self-damage and do not interfere with major functions.

His distress when they are removed seems clearly – though inexplicably – prompted by the knowledge that he will not be able to refrain from hurting himself. Yet he doesn't want to. It is a problem for all the mind experts to get their teeth into and they are obviously making a meal of it.

Was it a mistake to put the restraint on him in the first place? 'No,' Gary says. 'It was either that or keeping him asleep all the time with drugs.'

Phyl has started on the vacuuming. The children are downstairs, three of them in the playroom, the others around the house.

9.10 a.m.

The school bus arrives to take the children to school. 'The cattle truck,' Gary calls it. It is a large, battery-operated, closed-in van, with a few wooden seats inside and an elevating platform at the back, which everyone can just about squeeze on to.

They do not walk the short distance, because, in the event of one child being away from school, it would be impossible for one person to manage the rest alone, with Sandy moving at a snail's pace and Ronnie haring away after motor vehicles!

Nancy is agitated, biting her hand, clutching my arm. Gary has warned her before leaving the house that if there is any trouble at school, she will have him to answer to. She nodded calmly, but inside the bus her behaviour changes.

The school is something of a local showpiece, newly built, spacious and well-equipped (but with severe staff shortages, because of lack of money to pay them, one of the teachers complained). It takes children from that hospital, from another hospital and a few non-residents.

The Oakengates children are in different classes. Nancy's teacher, young and new to the school, looks distraught. Nancy had, in Gary's words, 'wrecked the classroom' a couple of days before. 'She really needs one-to-one all the time,' the teacher says. 'She is a danger to the other children. Yesterday she threw a toy push-chair across the room and hit another girl. The poor kid's head was pouring with blood.'

James's teacher, who had Nancy in her class for a while, backs this up. 'She is the most tantalizing, tormenting child. She will go for the helpless children who cannot defend themselves, without provocation.'

This is a new view of the little girl with the big brown eyes and the curly eyelashes. Outside Oakengates, it seems, it is she and not James who is Public Enemy Number One. She does not hit out much at Oakengates. A few mistakes like hitting Ronnie who could hit harder, seem to have cured her!

Gary has offered to come round to the school if she is proving too much of a handful, 'to sort her out'. Fifteen minutes after arrival, on our tour of the school, he is sent for. He takes her away and she returns silent and subdued. 'She's a funny kid,' he said to the teacher, 'because you are new, she is trying it on. She will push you to the limit to see how far she can go, but she knows who's boss.' The teacher looks unconvinced.

There is a surprising lack of liaison between hospital and school – surprising because they are so close, virtually on the same campus. The situation itself is not unusual.

There would surely be much to be gained from a nursing assistant going into school with the children each day, instead of dropping them at the door. She could find out what work teachers were doing with them and carry on with it at home. Participation by parents is usually encouraged but not, it appears, by nurses in parental roles, although senior staff at the hospital pay lip service to the idea.

It would not work, the staff insist at Oakengates. It has been tried in other places, but school staff resent the intrusion. Yes, they would love to know what the children are being taught, but not under sufferance . . . and two sides of the children's lives that could be mutually supportive, remain separate. A breakdown in communications somewhere.

BRIDGE HOUSE

There is little point in a detailed description of the day at Bridge House – it differs in only small ways from Oakengates and both differ little from life in your house or mine. Which is, of course, the strong point of the small Homes. To read about, they are boringly ordinary, which is just what the children need.

'You can come round and see what we do here in the mornings, by all means,' said Mr J, 'but cooking bacon and making tea here is much the same as anywhere else.'

The difference between the two Homes is mainly a matter of location. Bridge House is in a surburban street. They have had to involve themselves in the community, or live in isolation, which perhaps makes them closer to the ideal for this kind of Home.

It did not happen naturally. There was opposition to the house being used as a Home from, among other quarters, the local tenants' association, which is now their closest ally and includes the children on its outings.

Mr J went from door to door, inviting neighbours in for coffee and a chat. He contacted local firms, who willingly got involved and helped pay for garden play equipment and the record player which blares almost continually in one of the downstairs lounges.

The children – three mongol girls and two boys – are teenagers aged between thirteen and fifteen. The girls in particular are very capable, able to dress and wash themselves (even their hair, in the bath), toilet trained and capable of communication.

Karen took me on a guided tour of the house, pointing out her room (shared with another girl) with pop posters over the bed, personal effects around, her own wardrobe and cupboard. Karen, like the other children, attends a local special school, and Mr J has a vaguely parental relationship with staff there. The head teacher attends the three-monthly conferences on each child at the Home.

Karen has a boyfriend, attending the same school, but living at home, who calls regularly. 'He is buying me an engagement ring,' she said. 'I don't know why he bothers,' a member of staff said, 'they just fight all the time.'

There is little talk of programmes or training at Bridge House. The children join in with washing-up and, at weekends, help cook breakfast and make their beds. They do a little supervised laundry and clean their shoes every evening. Three girls and one boy will go to hostels when they reach sixteen, as did the older boy who came here with them three years ago and left last year.

The odd-man-out in the set-up is Gregory. He arrived from the hospital eighteen months ago and is much more dependent, non-communicating, possibly autistic. Now, there is a programme, worked out with the hospital psychologist for Gregory, written in detail and hung on the wall of his single bedroom. Behaviour modification is not mentioned, but the aim is to teach him to dress and wash himself, and use the toilet spontaneously.

The detailed programme is the result of a snag also encountered at Oakengates – the amazing fact that there are as many different ways to interpret the order to put on a jumper as there are people.

Mr J explained. 'At first I would just say "help him to get dressed", then "help him to put on his vest and jumper, then underpants and trousers". But everyone was doing it a little differently and it was confusing Gregory even more. We had to break it down into very small stages.'

Every day after school, while the other children are playing in the garden or listening to records, one staff member takes Gregory to his room and he goes through his undressing, washing, dressing programme. They report considerable success, but nobody holds high hopes of him reaching the stage of self-sufficiency the others have attained.

The girls tend to help look after him. They are sociable children and play together on swings and a climbing frame. They are enthusiastic telly-viewers. I sat through 'Crossroads' and 'Top of the Pops' with them and a nursing assistant one night. A very civilized evening, interrupted only by Karen bursting into tears and being reprimanded when her favourite group were not on, then Cindy blocking the view with indistinguishable impersonations of a go-go dancer, then of an elephant she saw on a trip to the zoo.

During the school holiday, they had gone out regularly as a group – by hospital transport to the zoo, the seaside, a stately home; on foot for a walk or to the park. Other days, selected children from the neighbourhood, like the family next door whose mother is a nursing assistant, had been in to play.

Here they part company with Oakengates. 'The Bridge House kids don't go to the hospital swimming-pool or join in hospital events.

They don't mix with mentally handicapped children,' one Oakengates helper said wryly.

The Oakengates six, on the other hand, had spent a lot of the holiday on outings with children from the hospital or at the rather grand, heated swimming-pool there. They had been lucky enough to have, for the first time, a team of young volunteers recruited through the hospital; enough to take them out almost every weekday on a one-to-one basis. A relief, too, for staff who face the same holiday trauma as parents. Bridge House had apparently not requested this sort of arrangement.

Each child at Bridge House has his or her own 'bank account'. Out of their 'pocket money' allowance each week, £1.70 is paid into this to cover outings and expenses and supplement the clothing allowance. This stands at £32, but is due for a large increase, and extra clothes can be taken from the hospital's central supply. Every day, each child is given 7p, counted out into their hands, to spend at the local sweet shop or save in a money box.

They line up to collect this, clutching purses, as if it were a King's Ransom. It can be partly withdrawn for bad behaviour and is treated very seriously. Except for Gregory, they are allowed to go singly along the road – a fairly busy one – to the shop. Instructions to wave to the butcher ensures the child has to be in the safe spot on the pavement – and the butcher apparently is friendly.

'We used to have a bit of trouble,' Mr J explained. 'They would choose something worth more than 7p in the shop and the woman there, out of kindness, would let them have it for what they had got. When we realized what was going on, we persuaded her not to. The whole point is for them to learn the value of money and how to count it.'

'I don't want the kids to get preferential treatment. They have to live in society as it is. They cannot be protected for ever. People say it is a bad idea to have normal children play with them, that they might tease them. As I see it, this is going to happen to them later on whatever we do. Within reason they might as well get used to it now. It is no good cushioning them.'

'The same goes with taking on staff. It would be easy to find someone who will be nice to them, but much harder to find someone who can be strict and tell them off when they need it. We have a very flexible staffing arrangement here. People come in when they are needed. I like staff who don't stand watching the kids. They are expected to show some initiative, to join in and do things with them.'

There is no talk of staff shortages at Bridge House, though they work to the same ratio system as Oakengates. The children, even Gregory, are simply less time-consuming. They are, though, what you might call a dying breed. There are now few children so mentally able living in hospitals. Future 'satellite' children are far more likely to be of the Oakengates ability level.

Conclusions

This is one possible path hospitals can take from the crossroads where they now stand – and many have already taken the first tentative steps. This is the hospital as resource-centre, housing its own population (and we will leave aside the arguments about who they should be) whilst administering and serving small satellite units within its catchment area.

It seems the best of both worlds. Without good social, medical and educational facilities nearby, an inefficient or unlucky Community Home could become as isolated as any old-style hospital. The central hospital can provide these services, but with the right staff and the right mix, the Home can still retain its comfort, homeliness and autonomy.

Everyone involved emphasizes the importance of the right mix of children. Some felt this sort of Home could accommodate more severely handicapped, even multiply handicapped, as long as you kept to one category of child and did not mix them. Others, but fewer, thought a mix of the physically handicapped and the relatively able would be ideal and mutually beneficial. I'm with them. The children at Bridge House seemed to enjoy having a less able boy to help, though those in the other Home were too self-involved, too severely handicapped, really, consciously to help their problem boy. But then he is in a different category, anyway. Who wants a bite or a punch for their trouble?

There are obvious queries. Is it fair to give Sandy a taste of something approaching family life, then plunge her back into the anonymity of a hospital ward when she does not make the grade? Isn't that even more cruel than leaving her there in the first place? Shouldn't it be a home for life, or another similar Home for over-sixteens be provided?

There is an element of being on trial for the children at Oakengates. It would be nice if, whether they passed or failed, they were assured of going on to a future as good as the present.

Staff as individuals are doubly important in this setting. The untrained people have to take more responsibility, use more initiative than their opposite numbers in hospital. There, everything is cut and dried; jobs and even permitted feelings, clearly defined.

The women at Bridge House in particular did not talk of seeing themselves as substitute mothers. One thought of herself as a combination of teacher and friend. 'I think too much fuss is made about these children missing someone who leaves. I used to think so, but I've watched people go and they forget them very quickly, as long as someone pleasant takes over.'

And another: 'It is hard to think of them as handicapped. They are just young children. Isn't that what every woman wants – children who never grow up?'

Initially I felt that the lack of house-parents – a couple actually living on the premises night and day – would detract from the homely feeling. But it didn't seem to. The night nurse was a familiar face (or two or three faces) to the children, too, and their routine was not changed by her presence. One charge nurse had had a spell of living in and did not feel anyone should be asked to do it.

'You are putting the nurse or house-parent into the situation that made the parents put the child in care in the first place, only magnified six times. You work better with these kids when you have regular breaks and come back fresh.'

And which of the two systems is best – near the hospital or truly in the community, miles away? I am inclined to plump for the advantages – to staff as well as residents – of the first, particularly with more handicapped children. But those in charge of the Home would have to make a continuous effort to become part of the community and not take the easy option of slipping back under the wing of the mother hospital.

These two places, sadly, are a drop in the ocean – and one may soon be put to different use anyway. It is three years since the last one opened and there are no plans by the hospital despite the admitted success – to open more. Why? Money, money, money! It costs more to run and staff a Community Home than to keep six children in a hospital ward.

Another factor is the widespread uncertainty about the future role of hospitals. Soon there may not be any children in hospitals to go out to satellite homes, so they would be superfluous.

In theory at least, the Social Services should soon be providing small units in the community for all children in their area needing permanent placement. Though senior hospital staff do not appear to be entirely convinced that this is imminent, neither are they prepared to rush in and spend money in this area themselves.

The nursing officer in charge of these two Homes pointed out that if Local Authorities fulfil their obligations speedily, none of the children, however limited, will go back to hospital. They should be placed in adult hostels or small Homes by the time they reach sixteen.

And, if they do go back to the hospital – where, incidentally numbers per ward are decreasing all the time – there will be the chance of going to a small community unit, 'when there is one to go to.'

3

Local Authority Provision – Life in the Community

'We are still learning, but there is tremendous enthusiasm. Some terrific ideas are emerging. The whole concept of care for the mentally handicapped is changing. I wish people would stop carping about what we have not done and look at the amount we have achieved in a short space of time.' So says a young – and enthusiastic – social worker, based in a city with approximately 3,000 mentally handicapped people needing some Local Authority help.

It is a good philosophy, but it does not build the hostels and the small community homes of which we have heard so much and seen so little, since the 1971 White Paper *Better Services for the Mentally Handicapped.*

On whose responsibility it should be to provide residential accommodation and care, the paper placed the ball firmly in the Local Authority's court. Ever since, they have been accused of not playing the game.

Take, for instance, the most sensitive subject – mentally handicapped children in hospitals. Nobody thinks they should be there, and the plan is, and has been for nearly a decade, to move them into small, home-like, family units run by the Social Services in the community. Such units are notable up and down the country by their scarcity or complete absence.

Many people and organizations working in this field believe that, rather than making recommendations, the government should set a firm date when children will no longer be admitted to or kept in hospital, forcing Local Authorities to accept their responsibility. As always, it is a question of finance. Social Services Departments invariably have desperate, diverse calls on their purses and rate-payers are none too keen to foot extra bills.

At least the mentally handicapped have become an area of major concern, a priority issue. There is much discussion, and plenty of imaginative ideas are emerging. The quantity lags sadly behind, but the quality so far is promising.

Hostels are still the main type of accommodation but there has been a gradual realization that they need not be the only way of providing it. Group Homes are increasingly popular. 'Digs' and multi-occupied private lodging houses are being used, although this method has developed an appalling reputation for poor meals, overcrowding and rogue landlords.

Brighter ideas being discussed at length – though hardly ever taken further – include sheltered housing (living alone with shared facilities and support services); 'cluster flats' with a warden on hand; intensively staffed hostels able to take the severely and multiply handicapped; hostels specially for the young-adult age group; fostering schemes, not only for children, but boarding-out adults with suitably interested families, willing to provide a taste of home life.

A lot of effort is being put into providing short-term care, particularly for under-sixteens, which should reduce the demand for permanent care – or at least postpone it. The enthusiasm mentioned by the specialist social worker I spoke to is no figment of the imagination. She and others like her spend a lot of time meeting parents' groups to find out their needs. There is a belief in sharing ideas with parents and other professionals.

They are willing to learn. Minds are not closed. Ideas are not set. Other people are not scorned. But all that does not build and staff hostels or provide anything like the amount of support residents, staff and parents need.

Joint funding has been a boon to Local Authorities, though again they have been criticized – for using it wrongly, or simply being too nervous to use it much at all.

This involves central government funds being transferred from the DHSS to Local Authorities to set up specific projects. It is intended as a pump-priming exercise. The financial support lasts up to five years, then the Social Services have to pick up the bill. Wary of landing themselves with large bills in the near future, they've tended to use the money for short-term projects or those with low running costs.

One way joint funding has been used successfully is to make grants to voluntary organizations wishing to set up Homes. Social workers liaise closely on such schemes, offering guidance, sometimes eventually taking over the running. Apart from adding an extra resource to their list, it provides a painless chance to monitor new and experimental schemes on a small scale with a view to running an enlarged version if it proves successful.

The pressure at the moment is for quantity of places, but of course the quality is desperately important, too. Here, they are having to learn as they go. Each place is new and highly individual. It will take a few more years to see an overall picture and reach conclusions.

Teams have been set up or individuals appointed in Social Service Departments to monitor standards in residential units and to offer guidance and support – managerial, moral and professional – to the people who run them. Different people are coming to work in residential care. It is no longer a poorly paid, dead-end job, but tends more and more to attract qualified 'career carers'.

There is a fairly generalized belief among those working for Local Authorities that hospitals can be made redundant – though not the skilled people who work in them – and they can efficiently take over the care of the mentally handicapped. It is just taking longer than anyone envisaged.

A Hostel

BOX TREES

Box Trees is three years old and purpose-built – one of the new breed of Local Authority hostels and it caters for twenty-five people. Places in these are quite sought-after by parents, 'Local Authority' tending to be synonymous in people's minds with 'community-based' and hostel being the word of the moment, conjuring up visions of freedom and independence.

Oddly enough, though, there is a growing, almost imperceptible swing among parents away from the 'hostels rule' notion, back to a preference for the 'Home', with its connotations of security and control.

But that's another story. Hostels are here to stay and for those people they suit, that's good news. They do not, by any stretch of the imagination, suit every mentally handicapped adult, in their present form. They tend to cater only for the sociable and relatively capable and, in theory at least, many are seen as an intermediate stage between hospital and group Home for a percentage of the people who come to them.

Box Trees, for instance, has a Minimum Care Unit attached – a large flat where five people can live in virtual independence from the main hostel, doing their own cooking, cleaning and washing.

The idea is for them to move on when they have mastered the skills of living independently, but they tend to get stuck in a bottle-neck in 'mini-care', because of the shortage of suitable outside accommodation. In any case, very few hostel residents, though capable of living with minimum supervision, have the potential to graduate to a flat or a group home.

Mrs L, the officer in charge of the hostel, is sure, though, that there are still many people in hospital who would benefit greatly from a hostel place – but there are not nearly enough to go round.

Most of the residents have come from local hospitals. Betty, in her forties, who now has a job as a cleaner in a Home for the elderly, came to the hostel from a group Home. She had been sent out to this group, with no training, after spending most of her life in hospital. Not surprisingly, the placement had broken down and she came to the hostel, where she is one of the success stories.

A few, like Jilly – a sweet-faced, deaf mongol in her thirties – came straight from home, when their parents died. Jilly, according to Mrs L, joined her hands and raised tearless eyes to heaven with a smile, to explain her mother's disappearance. She cannot talk. Despite thirty-five years of devoted care at home, she adapted almost at once and has struck up a close friendship with Stuart ('a real gentleman,' said Mrs L), less handicapped than herself and very protective towards her. She still has the gentle, dependent look that most of the others have long since had to jettison.

Mrs L was a teacher – first with normal children, then with the mentally handicapped – before going into residential care. Her husband also works in the same field. She has grown-up children and grandchildren and still retains a somewhat headmistressy attitude – more apparent to the staff than the residents, and to curious interlopers, like myself.

'You're always getting at me,' said one middle-aged resident, rushing away in tears, after being soundly questioned and reprimanded, about 'borrowing' another resident's necklace. I could understand her feeling, when I was reprimanded for pouring out, sugaring and stirring tea for a very gentle man with a broken leg, sharing my table.

'He is an adult, not a child,' she said coolly, amid excuses from me about him being incapacitated. 'He does not pour out tea with his leg,' she said.

She is appalled by the degree to which parents and the uninformed public deprive the mentally handicapped of their independence by doing everything for them. 'Many parents ruin their children's lives by making them totally dependent.'

Apart from two double rooms, all residents have single rooms with their own wardrobes and wash-basins. They are responsible for keeping these rooms clean and tidy themselves, but a quick tour with the senior care assistant showed that, while a few people are naturally tidy, a lot need reminding. And reminding is what they get, to the point of nagging. Staff are under instructions not to do it for them – though Wanda, the senior assistant, admits she helps Peter at the moment (the man with the broken leg, who was my downfall). The same goes for one of the men in 'mini-care' who has a factory job and has to leave at 6 a.m. 'You can't expect him to do his own room before he goes, can you?'

The self-sufficiency rule extends to laundry. There is a laundry room next to the kitchen, equipped with washing-machines, tumble dryer and iron. Each resident does his or her own laundry, some with reminders and supervision, others spontaneously. The training can be slow and tedious. Mrs L has battles with staff who tend to do the work for them, to hurry the process up.

There are two cooks and a kitchen assistant, plus two cleaners. They have to be willing to involve themselves with the residents, not just stick within the narrow definition of their jobs. Residents help maintain common areas on a rota system – there is, for instance, a list in the kitchen of people who wash up after breakfast and tea, each week.

The rest of the staff comprises Mrs L, her deputy (they were awaiting a replacement in a month's time when I was there, the previous one having left to start a short-term hostel), third officer and five care assistants.

One of these women works almost exclusively in a teaching capacity, taking groups of residents to the 'mini-care' unit to teach them simple tasks, like making a pot of tea and cooking their lunch. Not with a view to going out, simply as a useful skill. It is a job Mrs

L created, having noticed instinctive teaching ability in this woman, who has no training.

Mrs L has freedom to choose and deploy her staff as she wishes. Most are untrained but she finds it useful to have someone who is incidentally a nurse around the house. Otherwise, she says, she looks for people with understanding, liking for the residents and warmth. 'You have to be able to show affection for these people with a hug, rather than a polite hello or thank you.'

Box Trees stands at the furthest end of a slightly run-down road in a city suburb. On one side are ordinary dwellings, on the other a common and a patch of waste land, which, until the Council cleared it recently, had become a rat-infested dump.

They claim a good relationship with the neighbours. Residents have to walk the full length of the road to get their special bus to the adult training centre. The few who have jobs travel the same way – so neighbours get to know them.

Fear of jeopardizing this relationship made them send back to hospital, post haste, a young man who went in for exposing himself.

One of the younger girls, who took up throwing stones at passing cars, got a telling off and a sharp smack on the bottom from Mrs L – which seems to have cured her, though she does have her behaviour problems. In general, difficult people are simply not referred. Social workers are well aware of the range of acceptability.

What they don't get is the massive neighbourhood financial support afforded a similar but voluntary-run unit I visited. They don't ask, for one thing, but neither do people rush forward to offer help for something run by a statutory body. It is assumed that all their needs are well taken care of – which is not always true.

The building itself is on two floors. Downstairs is the dining-room, kitchen, laundry room, games room (full of jumble for an impending sale when I was there, but staff organize a weekend disco sometimes), a telephone booth for residents, one of two bathrooms (two baths, two toilets, one shower) and a television lounge, with a tiny kitchenette next door with an electric kettle for residents to make tea or coffee.

Upstairs are the bedrooms, a second bathroom unit and another television lounge – this time with colour set, so it is the most popular. The residents contribute to the rental of this set and are forbidden to fiddle with its knobs themselves.

There are no rules, staff are fond of telling you – this is a home.

In fact, there are rules and many of them, mostly governing acceptable behaviour. There have to be. It's just that they are not written down.

It is a functional, sparsely furnished and naked-looking place. Vinyl tiles on all floors, pale emulsion on all the walls. They have had only two rooms papered by the Local Authority in two years.

Only the absolute minimum of furniture was provided. Over the years, Mrs L has added bits and pieces given them by friends – pieces of carpeting in the games room and the hall, an ancient, battered settee in the entrance hall, a sideboard that has seen better days in the television lounge.

It gives it a homely look, she says. It also gives it a seedy, second-hand look in places. Mrs L and her husband, who works at another hostel, live in a flat on the premises. On her days off, another staff member will sleep in to be on call.

There are no set bed-times and the door seems to be ever-open. Mrs L says she knows of otherwise excellent establishments, where the adult residents come down to watch television in their night-clothes and at exactly 10 p.m. the plug of the set is pulled out, the lights go off and 'forty-year-old women who have been out to do a day's work are sent up to their beds like children'.

If residents are out at a club for the handicapped – as some of them are three nights a week – Mrs L has to wait up to see them safely in at 11 p.m. One 'mini-care' man goes to the local pub most nights, taking enough money for two pints of beer. Money is handed out 'as needed'.

'They don't understand money. They ask when they want some and they usually get it. Otherwise they would just spend it all at once,' Wanda explained. This seems to extend to those who go out to work and earn a full wage. The pub-goer has a factory job, which he has held for years.

Mrs L usually does her last checks at midnight. It is not inconvenient, she says, because she lets her dogs out then. She has two dogs and several cats, which roam around freely and are fed (the cats) on left-overs collected for them in a special dish after meals. They were useful when the rats were running riot on the adjoining land.

Thursday 5 p.m.

Most of the residents are home and seated around tables for four in the dining-room. It is stew for the evening meal, followed by apple crumble for those not on diets and an apple or orange for those who are. A surprising number are on diets – and not all of them are too happy about it. After all, a couple of staff members are fairly substantial themselves.

The evening meal is usually a little lighter than this, as most residents – those at adult centres – get a cooked midday meal. But a bread strike has made snacks harder to come by than main meals, for the moment.

On duty are Mrs L and Wanda, who has come in with a heavy cold, because of staff shortages. Mrs L is looking tired. She has been on duty since 8 a.m. and still has office work to do. She takes her husband some dinner from the kitchen to their flat, comes back and sits down to share a pot of tea with Clare and Peter.

Clare, just over twenty, is the hostel's 'naughty girl'. It was she who threw stones at passing cars, and later in the evening she instigates an argument with one of the older women in the television lounge. Over the tea-table, there is a typical outbreak. Clare wants a pudding, but she is on a diet. Mrs L makes her take back the one she has helped herself to from the serving counter. She shouts, slams cutlery around the table, threatens to run away.

Nobody reacts, except Mrs L moving the excessively gentle Peter, for his own safety, to the next table. 'She is doing this for your benefit, I'm afraid,' she says. There is another Clare, a pretty, dark girl. Introducing her, Wanda explains, 'This is "Good" Clare, the other one is "Bad" Clare.' Not, fortunately, in 'Bad' Clare's hearing.

There is no lack of affection for the girl, however – rather the opposite. 'She's a poor little thing, really,' Wanda says. 'When I was in the West Indies on holiday I sent her a card, just for herself. I often ring her up when I'm off duty to let her know there is someone interested. She has no one of her own, you see.'

Hugh, the factory worker, goes into the kitchen to collect his sandwiches for the next day. Mrs L is concerned that, despite bread shortages, he must get 'enough for a working man'. There is a minor upheaval, as Bobby, another middle-aged man who has just found a job despite a life-time in hospital, goes in for his sandwiches, then comes out looking upset.

The cook follows him out. 'You think Hugh is having something on his sandwiches that you aren't, don't you?' A small worried nod. 'It's not true. When he has fish, you have half a tin each. You get exactly the same, except when it's cheese, because you don't like cheese.'

The matter seems to be settled. Bobby lights up another cigarette and sits smoking quietly. Only a few of the residents smoke. Betty, the ex-hospital patient and cleaner extraordinary, is one who does. It is her big failing. A few small holes in her bedspread bear witness to the fact that it is not confined to the public rooms. Mrs L would rather it was, though there is no set rule.

Betty arrives late for tea, because she has been making coffee for one of the men in the 'mini-care' unit. Mrs L reprimands her. 'You mustn't wait on him. You've been out at work, too.' But Betty is a compulsive worker. A thin, wiry woman, with a lined, worn face, she mopped floors and helped nurses when she was at the hospital. She is just as efficient at the old people's home. An astounded matron rang Mrs L to tell her that Betty even turns the tables over and washes underneath them. 'And she's kind to the old people, too.'

Raymond, whom Mrs L has described as 'the handsomest young man in the area' arrives late, as well. He has just come in and explains, very articulately, that he has been looking in the shops on his way home. He is tall, fair, good-looking – and looks and sounds very normal. He appeared to be forming a relationship with one of the girls, but has cooled off since starting work and meeting new people.

It is hard to ascertain a general hostel attitude to relationships between the sexes. The only firm friendship, which everyone regards as 'sweet' is between Jilly and Stuart, another unobtrusive, well-liked mongol in his thirties.

One woman is planning to get married and has approached the local vicar, with her fiancé, a man she met at a club for the mentally handicapped. 'She's feeble-minded more than mentally handicapped, and she is too old to have children,' Mrs L points out. She is nagging the Council to find a flat nearby for the pair, where they can be supervised by the hostel.

A few of the younger women are on the pill – some because they were when they arrived from hospital and are still under the wing of the hospital consultants; others because Mrs L thought it better to be safe than sorry, with them travelling freely to work and around the neighbourhood. 'Better than put a girl through the trauma of abortion, but we do not automatically put every girl on the pill.'

There is a system – liberated for hostels, Mrs L insists – of mixing the sexes on each corridor of bedrooms. Usually there is one wing for the girls and one for the boys. Mrs L reasons that shrouding the women in mystery is bound to intrigue the men and lead to the occasional Peeping Tom.

'This way, they get used to seeing a girl going down the hall in her nightie. It soon ceases to excite curiosity.'

The bulk of the residents are middle-aged and fairly staid anyway. Mrs L deliberately wanted 'a core of people in their thirties and forties, who are more settled to build the hostel around. She has little faith in the theory that young people adapt best to the independence of hostel life.

'If they have been in hospital since early childhood, as a lot of my people have, they are no less institutionalized – and they are, on average, far more likely to be disruptive and aggressive. We have young people now, but they came after the older ones had settled in and done the groundwork of making it a home.'

6 p.m.

Except for the late-comers, most people have drifted off. Some have gone to have baths. They usually have a bath twice a week, on a rota.

A young girl goes off to do her ironing. She has a father and two sisters who visit her regularly, but the father never, ever takes her home. Mrs L muses a little about the oddness of this.

Wanda has joined her at the table for a cup of tea and together they look through some clothes handed in for the jumble sale, to see if there is anything respectable that will fit one of the girls. It explains why some of the girls, though neat and tidy, have a distinct 1960s look about their clothes. One of the older women is wearing a pair of trousers that were Mrs L's. Trendy they are not. The jumble sale is to raise money for extras, like the summer holiday. Last year they went to Guernsey.

Hugh, the factory worker, needs a new pair of shoes. 'I hear you split your shoe,' Mrs L says. Hugh shakes his head. 'But you told me yourself,' she insists. They talk at cross-purposes for a while, then all is explained. 'I didn't *do* it,' he says. 'It happened.' They decide to ask Hugh's sister, 'a good friend to Box Trees' to get a pair from the warehouse where she works and bring some more for other residents to try at the same time.

Each care assistant has special responsibility for a group of residents, to keep a check on points like the need for new clothes or shoes, getting a haircut, whether they are putting on weight or losing too much. Residents' names are picked out of a hat for allocating and changed every couple of months. 'If they could pick, there would be some people all the staff would want, and others nobody would touch.' Outside the dining-room door, a big man with a hang-dog expression is standing, waiting.

'He's loitering again,' Wanda says, her sunny temper evaporating suddenly. The culprit is brought in and stands speechless and anxious before the two women. What is he doing? Why is he standing there? Hasn't he been told before, they demand. It turns out he is waiting for his bus fare for tomorrow. More questions: What time is it? When is the bus fare usually given out? Has he tidied his room? He hasn't tidied his room. He is told to do so – *now*. He shuffles away: a large, lumpy, sad, middle-aged child. Not, I presume, one of the popular names out of the hat.

In the hall, Don is sitting on the settee, watching the door. Mrs L tells him amiably – she treats Don with almost exaggerated respect – that he should not be there, the hall is only for people who are waiting.

'I *am* waiting,' he says, 'I'm waiting for my visitors.'

Don is an unusual case. Mrs L firmly believes he shouldn't be there at all and has him on a strict diet as a first step to getting him into a group home or a place of his own. She has also fixed up dental appointments to deal with dreadfully neglected teeth and is taking him for interviews at workshops for the disabled, not the mentally handicapped.

On a previous midday visit, I had shared a table with Don and a temporary woman resident. (Staff and residents who are not out during the day, for whatever reason, get a cooked meal.)

Don had expounded knowledgeably on a variety of topics from medicine to cave drawings. Yet, because his mother refused to send him to a special school, he was only educated for a year as a young child and a further year in his teens. He is now in his forties and cannot read or write, though Mrs L is convinced he has the potential and is trying to get him into a literacy scheme.

Where did he accumulate this wealth of knowledge, I wondered? 'Television,' he said. 'I used to watch it a lot when I was at home with my mother.'

Don's mother (one of Mrs L's over-protective problem parents) devoted her life to him. His father, he said, was just the opposite. Mrs L rushed in to defend the man, saying he was only far-sighted and tried to give Don some independence. Whatever the reasoning when Don's mother literally dropped dead, he was alone in the world and had to be found residential care urgently. He had gone to an old people's home, where he helped the nurses, and then was moved to Box Trees.

He likes it there, the people are friendly, he says. But he joins with a reasonable amount of enthusiasm in the scheme to rehabilitate him. He wouldn't mind a flat of his own, he thinks. 'It would depend. . . .'

'Better have a bath before I go to that centre,' he told Mrs L over lunch. 'I don't want to let my Mum down.' Mrs L looked uncertain how to interpret that. 'You, I mean,' he added mischievously. She looked even more uncertain.

Several of the residents call Mrs L by her Christian name. It is something she encourages. And it is only fair to say that whilst I found her attitude at times distancing – and that may come across here – there were frequent displays of spontaneous affection for her from residents.

She obviously cares, and is prepared to back that up with time and attention, and a lot of respect for individuality. The residents of Box Trees are definitely people, not cases, and they are encouraged to think of themselves as very capable people.

Don was talking about a cousin, one of the few relatives who visits him. 'She is a bit like me – only she's not backward.'

'I don't want you to say that again,' Mrs L told him. 'You are not backward.'

7 p.m. – The television room

The dozen straight, armless chairs lining the walls are taken and a small, cheerful man, comes in and sits cross-legged on the carpet.

Like half-a-dozen other residents, he came from the closest mental handicap hospital and they all know each other. 'Bad' Clare and Greta, the bride-to-be, are prone to sudden, unexplained verbal eruptions towards each other, which everyone else ignores.

Normally, half the residents go out to a local club for the handicapped, but as they have to walk and it is very foggy, they are not being allowed to go today. There are three regular clubs a week. The only entertainment facility on the premises, apart from television, is the games room and it is not used much. Some hostels organize more recreational facilities, particularly dancing, Mrs L says, but it depends on staff and she is not the disco type.

Greta is a plump, rather sullen-looking woman in her fifties. She talks eagerly about her wedding plans, but certainly with no awareness of doing anything unusual. Why should she? The idea of two mentally handicapped people getting married and living as happily ever after as anyone else is no longer revolutionary to the professionals involved with them. With increased community care and independent living, it is something we will all get used to in the future. Will Greta be able to cope with all that housework and housewifery? 'Yes,' she said. 'I looked after my father till he died.'

Greta's story is one of those Dickensian horror tales from the bowels of the subnormality hospitals. At the age of fourteen – one of a large, and what would now be called disadvantaged, family – she stole a vest worth eleven pence and three farthings. She was sent to a hospital and did not emerge again until a few years ago, when relatives took her out to nurse her dying father.

She did a job that could not be faulted and, when her father died two years ago, was again homeless and was taken into Box Trees as an emergency admission. Now, Greta is getting what she should have been given forty years ago, the chance to lead a normal life – with a little help from her friends.

The room is unsupervised. Mrs L comes in briefly to say something to Jilly, who can hear very little. Jilly, misunderstanding, leaps up and sits on the floor to let us have her chair. She is re-seated, looking very confused.

A little later, Wanda comes in. She has been round to see the baths are going well and distributed soap, where needed, from stores. Another couple are sitting together, holding hands and kissing ostentatiously when anyone glances their way. Which isn't often.

Most people prefer the television. 'A new love affair,' Wanda said. 'How sweet,' said Mrs L when she told her later.

7.30 p.m. – the dining-room

It's a staff coffee break – all two of them – and four residents have joined them. Not for a drink, though. Their supper is at 8 o'clock, when there is a milky drink, cake or biscuits and money for the next day, distributed as needed.

Roy, 35 and ex-hospital, is explaining to me – and his conversation is hard to understand – that he cannot go out alone because he once had a traffic accident. Mrs L hastens to put the record straight. He can go out almost any time, as long as she knows where he is. He goes out every day. He takes her dog for a walk.

'But my sister . . .' Roy begins, hesitantly, before being out-voted. His sister worries about him and discourages him from going out alone, Mrs L says. She also brings him chocolates, when he is on a diet.

The responsibility finally for who goes where belongs to Mrs L. She can think of only one girl who is likely to run away – and she runs home. She is not allowed out without other, responsible residents with her.

Betty arrives down, a cigarette in her mouth. She has had a lovely bath, she says, and scrubbed the baths out. She has washed her hair and plainly can't do a thing with it. Mrs L says she must go to the local hairdresser who deals with all the residents, and have a perm before the weekend. Betty has been invited to a staff party at work, which seems, superficially, to answer one worrying question – whether she is accepted by workmates.

Alice arrives, handbag over her arm, a scrap of paper in her hand with a number written on it. It is the number of the hospital where her 82-year-old father is seriously ill. Quite how ill, she obviously does not realize and she talks of going home to look after him.

Alice came to the hostel on a temporary basis when he was taken to hospital – another wrong placement, Mrs L feels. 'She is mentally ill, not handicapped. You can tell just by looking at her, but there are so many cases where the boundaries are blurred and it is hard to know which category they fit into. Anyway, there are even fewer hostel places for the mentally ill.'

There *is* something different about Alice. She is painfully thin, almost anorexic. On my previous visit, she ate nothing but a slice of beef off her dinner plate claiming she hated the rest. Tonight, she failed to come down for tea, and someone sent to fetch her brought back the answer that Alice was not hungry. It was not forced on her.

She speaks with perfect clarity – a lot of the residents are hard to understand – but refers to herself as 'me'.

'Me bought Dad a present for his birthday,' she said, getting out a boxed tie. 'He's 82 tomorrow.'

Her own age is hard to guess. She could be anything between thirty and sixty. 'Dad' is actually her step-father, which has not diminished her devotion. She worked for twenty years before giving up her job to look after him. She wants someone to help her phone the hospital, because she has trouble getting through to thc right ward. Wanda helps and, a few minutes later, she is back, smiling. She is going to visit him next day.

Her moods swing. The previous day I had seen her approach one of the dogs, pat and kiss it, then five minutes later, slap it on the nose. One of the cats was even less fortunate. Without any warning or reason, Alice bit its ear and hung on to the terrified animal when staff tried to unclench her teeth.

Back in the dining-room, Alice hums a tune, gives one of the younger girls – who looks worried about it – a few affectionate pats on the shoulder, and picks up the black cat. She begins to stroke the animal, cooing in its ear.

There is a sharp in-take of breath all round, but nobody moves.

'If you bite that cat's ear,' says Mrs L, sounding as if she means it, 'I will personally bite yours.'

8.10 p.m.

With apologies for seeming rude, but with undisguised relief, Mrs L sees me to the door. She has been on duty for twelve hours now, and is feeling the strain, and she is not the sort of person who will leave you to your own devices and take it easy.

The door is unlocked and we meet two men on their way in. Don's cousins have finally made it, an hour late. Mrs L does not diguise her irritation too well either. So far, there have been no set visiting hours – but she is going to introduce some, she says.

Conclusions

Everyone's fear about hostels is that they will rapidly turn into small institutions, as rigid as the hospitals they were set up to replace; that they may end up functioning as self-contained islands, which will make it irrelevant whether they are in the middle of a built-up area or the depths of the country.

It is easy to be in the community without being part of it, as people living in high-rise flats who have never met their neighbours will tell you.

Much depends on the people picked to run the hostels, for they have a greater degree of autonomy than is possible in a bigger unit, certainly in the cumbersome hierarchy of a hospital.

It makes finding the right people – and monitoring and helping them – vitally important. It is all very new and there are sure to be mistakes made, but the fact that everyone concerned seems aware of the pitfalls must be a good sign.

But what of Box Trees? First, it is not the free-and-easy home-from-home the staff suggest. That would be a lot to hope for in a centre catering for twenty-five people, with a fair number of problems between them. I would like to see smaller numbers in hostels, but then size is often decided by the economics of the situation, i.e. small units would be relatively expensive to run. Also, people with experience of hostels will tell you that small numbers, say a dozen people, make for personality clashes, because people who do not get on cannot easily avoid each other.

The hostel is not intended as a home for life for everyone. It is also a training centre, aiming to make all residents more self-sufficient and a few capable of moving on. This shows.

There is a certain classroom feel about the place. Meal times, for instance, tend to be training sessions. It may be necessary, but it is not very relaxing. This may sort itself out in time, when the group for whom it will inevitably become a home for life, have become more established. Money permitting, a separate training hostel would prove less disruptive for permanent residents.

I couldn't help comparing it with Chadwick House, a voluntarily-run home for thirty similarly handicapped adults, and finding it lacking. Not because of the setting, the food or the furniture but because of vaguer things, like attitudes and atmosphere. The definition of giving independence and treating people as adults seems confused. Ordinary social niceties, giving someone a helping hand as you might do with a perfectly normal adult, are frowned on as 'babying'. Yet in more basic ways, they are treated as children. Not being allowed, or taught to handle their own money, for instance – even the relatively able people.

Staff at the hospital I visited talked of patients being sent out to the freedom of hostels and asking to come back because they were bored, with nothing to do in the evenings and at weekends.

They were not totally unprejudiced, but it is easy to see how the hostel can appear socially limited, when games, discos, clubs and outings have been laid on, virtually in your own back yard.

Instigating a social life for residents is another job that falls to the officers in charge of the hostels – and varies with their initiative and enthusiasm. Ideally the residents should join in community events, moving as freely about the pubs, clubs, theatres and bingo halls as anyone else in the neighbourhood. In practice, they would not always be acceptable, nor would they necessarily enjoy it. So, it is up to Social Services departments to lay on some programme of suitable activities; at the moment they are mainly provided by voluntary groups.

Obviously hostels are here to stay, but they are not the be-all and end-all of community provision. Far from it.

They are a step in the right direction, but there are lots more routes to be explored – and problems to work out before anyone sits back and decides they have solved the problem.

Group Homes

NO. 35 AND THE CHERRIES

Brian and Michael are twenty-eight-year-old twins, sociable, capable, opinionated. They live, with two other young men, at No. 35 in a Group Home – that is, a council house, which they pay for with their own allowance or wages.

They live alone and do their own shopping, cooking, cleaning and socializing. They have a dog. Apart from the social worker who pops in a few mornings a week on his way to work and weekly to collect the rent, they are as independent as their neighbours. There is no telephone. The only safeguard for crisis is the address of the Social Services office which set up the Home, half a mile away. None of the four men has ever lived without either parents or supervisors before.

The concept of Group Homes is no longer new. It began as part of the great hospital exodus in the early Seventies, when councils, hospitals and voluntary bodies were looking around for less institutional ways of providing accommodation for the mentally handicapped.

As always, cost came into the reckoning – and you cannot find a much cheaper way of providing a home than renting or buying an ordinary house and letting the residents pay their own way and be their own cooks, cleaners and nurses.

It presupposes a fairly advanced grasp of the skills of everyday living, which is one reason why Group Homes have always been seen as a mere drop in the whole pool of residential places.

The supposition could be erroneous. Iris Cawley, who was involved in the setting up of an early and much studied Group Home, The Cherries, in Slough, feels that the idea could be extended to the severely handicapped, as long as the ability range was mixed within each home.

In The Cherries (built by Slough MENCAP and handed over to Buckinghamshire County Council), IQs ranged from 80 down to 37. In the two years that Mrs Cawley was involved with the Home, the amazing thing, she says, was that there were no problems.

'My phone number was painted on a wall by the telephone for emergencies but the only call I got was for advice when the bath plug came away from the chain it was attached to. The more able help the less able and enjoy doing so – that is what people overlook. Girls, in particular, denied maternity, long to look after people, almost like being a nurse. We underestimate mentally handicapped people terribly.'

The only essential requirement she feels, is 'clubability' – being able to get on with other people – and a relatively high IQ is no guarantee of that.

'That is the first basic essential which probably cannot be taught. I think they should also be able to take care of their personal hygiene and know when to change and wash their clothes to keep themselves in reasonable order. They don't have to be able to cut their own toenails. One of the other residents may help with that or a chiropodist can call.'

Michael and Brian's social worker, Mr O, is not totally in agreement with this view. He sees very few of his clients as candidates for such independent living.

He likes to take them straight from home, when they have some idea of what a family unit is like and haven't become institutionalized by hospital or hostel routine. 'Mind you, some people who have lived at home with protective parents for thirty years can be pretty institutionalized, too.' So Mr O ideally prefers dealing with younger people.

The twins in fact were at a hostel in the city for eighteen months, having lived at home most of their lives. Their elderly mother's illness had proved the final straw to a series of family problems, which had precipitated them into residential care.

The hostel had not suited them. 'Mrs L [the Warden] was too bossy' Michael – recognizable from his brother by two missing teeth – explained. 'She said we were too good for the place.' A delighted laugh. He laughs a lot and comments on events and questions with great enthusiasm. Brian is a bit more serious, a hard worker and probably the resident organizer, though Mr O insists that this is a completely democratic set-up.

It was Brian who was most adversely affected by hostel living. He has fits – which he appears to cope with, though he has not registered with a doctor – and they became severe during his spell there. All in all, it was thought that they would settle in a Group Home and rather than try to fit them into one already existing in the city, they were made the nucleus of a new one and two more compatible people sought.

Compatibility is the keynote. There must not be personality clashes or the scheme could collapse. Nor is there any question of simply moving four people to the house without their agreement.

The idea was discussed with Michael and Brian, then, when they showed interest, with their parents, who also liked the plan. The twins were brought over to see the house and to look around the area, on the opposite side of town from their own home.

When they seemed completely satisfied, they were given the keys, told to bring their parents over, come and go as they pleased and move when they were ready.

The twins moved in at the earliest possible moment. 'It's great,' Michael beams. 'We can do what we like. No one to boss us around.'

The third man to move in is no longer there. Problems are hinted at. He took his freedom too literally, it would seem, for a Group Home. There was a girlfriend involved. He has since got married and he and his wife live in a flat, with supervision.

Mr O points out that if Michael and Brian felt they would like to move on to even greater independence like a flat, it could be arranged. But No. 35 is their home for as long as they want it – unlike some authorities where the first Group Home acts as a kind of half-way house, getting residents used to the idea and they are then moved on to another permanent one. That, he feels – and I am sure he is right – is very unsettling.

There is a compatible quartet settled in the house now. Billy, whom I failed to meet, because he goes out a lot, walking his dog or to a club for the handicapped held in a nearby school, has a factory job. Andrew is shy and silent and a little lazy. That he manages to live unsupervised surprised me.

He lived at home all his life before coming here, not even attending an adult centre or sheltered workshop during the day. Now he goes daily to 'a sort of social centre'. His social worker says: 'He doesn't do any work there, but he meets people and he has made some friends. It is more to get him out of himself than anything. Left to his own devices, he will be happy to stay in his room playing his records all day, or even in bed. That is one of my reasons for calling in the mornings. Standards can start to slip.'

Andrew's mother lives nearby and he goes home for the weekend sometimes. Billy too lived at home previously and his mother has taken it on herself to keep an eye on the boys, calling in once a week to see that everything is in order. 'She is very useful and can report any problems,' Mr O said. 'If she didn't do this, we might have to have someone call on a regular basis to keep an eye on cleaning and things. You don't know. There are no rules for a place like this, no absolutes. You see how it goes, what is needed, and play it by ear.'

The men have their own keys and are free to come and go as they please, night and day. In fact, except for Billy, the others do not socialize much in the evenings. 'We go for a walk sometimes,' Michael said, 'or back to the hostel to see our friends.'

All four of them travel by bus and are fairly expert on the city's bus routes. Brian and Michael work at a car wash, not in the open market and not paying a full wage. It is sheltered work, employing psychiatric patients, but not many of the mentally handicapped.

'I think the twins were just lucky,' Mr O explained. 'When they left school, there were no vacancies at the Adult Training Centre, so they were found a place at the car wash. We have offered to try and find them an outside job, something less monotonous, but they don't want to move. They are happy where they are.'

Number 35 cost the Social Services £2,500 to set up. That paid for redecorating and furnishing. Each resident pays £8 a week to cover rent, rates, heating and lighting. This comes out of their wages or allowances. They handle their own finances.

Each individual buys and cooks his own food (except that the twins operate as a unit in the kitchen) supplemented by occasional goodies from parents and even pies from a neighbour who has taken them under her wing. Andrew does not cook elaborate meals, but his mother made a point of teaching him simple cookery at home. Billy owns a slow-cooking electric 'crock-pot'. He puts on his meal in the morning and it is cooked when he gets home.

The twins pride themselves on their culinary skills and always do a Sunday roast and bacon and egg breakfasts at weekends, though it is corn-flakes and toast during the week. They were planning a special spread for the following Sunday with their parents invited.

Other methods of operation have been tried in different places, like having one person at home all day, dealing with cooking and cleaning while the others go out to work or an adult centre. It is virtually putting him in charge, creating a warden and Mr O says he has seen it lead to a 'destructive situation'.

Certainly I have seen it, in another Group Home, lead to a micro-institution with rules more rigid than any hospital, imposed by the oldest resident who resented 'his' meals being left uneaten and 'his' rooms left untidy. A sort of manic-housewife syndrome that could end in mutiny.

That and a tendency for the weaker residents to become over-dependent on the group 'leader' – which I think probably happens anyway, even in a 'democratic' Group Home.

It is a three-bedroom house, the twins sharing the largest room. This standard size house can cause problems, combined with the standard number of four residents. The Social Services aim always for a house with two downstairs rooms, planned as a dining and sitting-room, but if necessary, one can be converted to a fourth bed-room. Even residents who have come from a crowded hospital ward soon develop territorial instincts, they have found, and want their own space and possessions.

The neighbourhood is important, they have discovered by trial and error over the years. A Group Home set up on an estate populated with problem families had to be closed because the residents were teased and tormented to danger point by local youths. Streets inhabited almost entirely by elderly folk with equally elderly prejudices are not ideal, nor are the bustling, self-involved 'young families only' Avenues and Closes.

No. 35 is, from a population viewpoint, perfect. A street of council houses, but in a quiet, middling suburb. A mixture of older people and families.

Mr O introduced the residents to neighbours as unselfconsciously as possible, trying not to make a big issue of it, when they were in the 'looking it over' stage with the house.

'I feel it is best when you have the residents there with you,' he says. 'If you go knocking on doors and telling them that mentally handicapped people are moving in next door, they get all sorts of funny ideas. When they meet them they realize they are ordinary people, no threat.' Nobody has complained – except for a little problem in the early days when Andrew played his records too loud and too late. The elderly lady next door asked him not to. That is all ironed out now and it is the sort of thing that could happen with any new neighbour.

It goes without saying really that a Group Home must be near to shops and bus routes and within walking, or short bussing, distance of someone in authority who can sort out problems. I would have imagined a telephone was essential, but Mr O says they cannot get one installed unless it is a pay phone with right of access to the rest of the neighbourhood. That would be, he points out, a potentially dangerous situation. He tells them not to let in strangers and worries a little about the possibility of them meeting and bringing home unscrupulous people. Such are the perils of freedom.

The twins took me on a conducted tour, with Andrew hanging back shyly. Their bedroom is clean but cluttered and untidy, with all sorts of oddments piled on chests and wardrobes. There is a religious picture on the wall, another general print, hanging upside down, because the cord has broken, cardboard keys from a relative's twenty-first birthday over Michael's bed.

Despite pleas that the missing Billy might resent such an intrusion on his privacy, they usher me into his room next-door. It is much tidier with a tea set, for some reason, arranged neatly atop a chest.

'If he comes in now, we'll tell him we've got him a girlfriend for the night,' said Brian, displaying a very normal sense of ghastly schoolboy humour. The twins are very acceptable anywhere, Mr O had said, without condescension. They had thought of separating them in case they became too dependent on each other, but had decided against it.

Downstairs, the two main rooms are adequately but sparsely furnished. Still after six months' residency, no sign of homeliness except for two small pictures in the dining-room, one belonging to Billy, one to Andrew. The furniture is standard Social Service issue – armless upholstered chairs so that a lighted cigarette could not become trapped (although in fact none of the four here smoke), flame-proof curtains and furnishing fabrics, an electric fire. There are electric heaters in the bedrooms and all heating comes out of the basic rent money, but there seems little risk of this costing the council a fortune. It was a chilly night, but nobody had turned on any heating.

The kitchen is roomy for the size of the house and the boys claim not to come to blows over all wanting to cook at once on one stove.

They were initially delivered two refrigerators, by mistake, but now the second one has been taken back – and they are missing it. Since they each buy their own food and milk separately, one is not enough they feel. By their choice, nothing is delivered and mostly they shop each day.

Do they ever run out of anything? No, they keep an eye on things to see when they are getting low and if they haven't got something they walk up the road to the shop, they say.

It is not an 'Ideal Home' kitchen. It suffers from the untidiness inherent in any kitchen shared by four people – and men – but it is not a shambles. A dog bowl with a half finished doggy meal stands just inside the door. Billy's dog sleeps out in a kennel in the garden when they are at work and at night, but when it is cold or wet, they let him stay in the kitchen.

Nobody objects to the dog – they were asked – but Mr O points out that is fortunate they did not have a pet each. The early resident, who has left, had mice which escaped and were eaten by the cat next door, causing a lot of distress all round.

'Look at the floor,' Brian said. 'It has to be washed every day.

You can't keep it clean. My sister had these tiles and she had to get rid of them. We are going to buy some mats to cover them.'

The pale matt tiles in kitchen and hall do indeed present a cleaning problem and Brian worries most about it. He comes into his own when talking about keeping the place up to scratch. He gets up at around 6 a.m. every Saturday (the twins are early risers every day, often having to call the others), washes his clothes, has a bath and sees to household laundry like towels and the net curtains too. Each man does his own washing.

There is a small back garden and a lawn-mower and tools inside the back door. The front garden has not been touched yet.

Don't they have a rota, I wondered, so that everyone can take share of the general work?

A small, indignant eruption from Brian. 'A list? We had a list at the hostel. I didn't like it. I know what has to be done. I don't need a list. When our Mum was in hospital, I did all the housework at home.' But does *everyone* know what has to be done? Don't they have to remind some people? Two sets of eyes turn towards Andrew, and Michael, laughing, gives him a playful nudge. Quarrels are minor ones, over which television channel to watch on the black and white set, for instance. The Social Services stopped putting radios in their houses because of disagreements over which station to have on.

The residents have their own radios and record players. Michael and Brian say they shop for their own clothes, without help, going into town to buy what they need. From the look of them, this is one area where they fall down. Both wore a strange assortment of old tatty shirts, jumpers and baggy pants, with buttons missing and big holes in the sleeves. Working clothes, admittedly, but nevertheless – tactful supervision would help. Sewing is one skill Brian and Michael have not mastered.

Something else that might have helped in this area is having a few women about. Mrs Cawley certainly thinks so. She believes that mixing the sexes is essential, not least because 'women get pleasure in bringing order out of chaos. It is unusual for men to like sweeping or dusting, but women often positively enjoy home-making and ironing and sewing'.

'I've no doubt that homes with women are tidier, warmer and just more homely. The all-male ones become a kind of barrack – and that has the added effect of making the men want to stay out as much as possible.'

An old-fashioned view of woman's role, but then mentally handicapped women are unlikely to have had their consciousness raised.

There was no definite plan to make No. 35 a single-sex establishment. There were just no girls ready, willing and able to be part of the quartet. The twins say they wouldn't mind girls sharing. It amuses them a bit. None of the men has a girlfriend. They are not discouraged, but Mr O admits that steady relationships, with the girl being brought home, can cause friction.

Another advantage of mixing the sexes, according to Mrs Cawley, is the safety of the girls. Although there was never any threatening behaviour towards any of the residents at The Cherries, despite its being situated on a big estate next to a working man's club, she still feels the presence of men might deter the rare drunk with evil intent.

'We are attracted to the opposite sex. We make more effort to look our best in their company. It is a more natural arrangement. You don't get sexual promiscuity. The home unit tends to be regarded as a family. The relationships are similar to those you get with a mixed group of students sharing a house.' Nevertheless, two of The Cherries' residents did get married and move to live in a flat nearby, with the blessings of everyone concerned.

The Cherries was purpose-built for twelve people, an atypically large number for a Group Home. People do tend to move through it to smaller homes or flats, too. Indeed there are people who would, because of the size, think of it more as a small, unsupervised hostel.

During Mrs Cawley's involvement with the Home, however, there was never a full quota. Residents arrived gradually, the first nucleus of four (three women and one man, aged between nineteen and thirty-six) coming from a hospital. Not the ideal starting-point, according to Mrs Cawley, 'because they have been so used to being told what to do or having it done for them'. The perfect group would have been, she insists, teenagers straight from home, with parental support in the background.

But Slough parents, like most, suffer from a reluctance to let their children go, until absolutely necessary – i.e. when they die – which may be too late. They are no longer acceptable – nor are parents here to help them settle.

'The absolute refusal of parents to think ahead,' is what Mrs

Cawley calls it (and she has a mentally handicapped teenager of her own).

All prospective Group Home dwellers spent two months training at a hostel and several trial weekends at the house – 'to get the feel of the place and to get to know people'. One of the big benefits of this has been learning about money. On a few occasions, money budgeted for the whole weekend was spent on Saturday leaving little in the larder for Sunday. No one in authority interfered and the residents concerned, having learnt the hard way, never made the same mistake again.

'Weekenders', as well as permanent residents, had to attend a meeting with a social worker after the evening meal had been eaten and the tidying done every Monday. It was the only curb on their freedom. At these group discussions, problems were thrashed out and solved – by the residents themselves. Mrs Cawley: 'The social worker would say, for instance "What shall we do about the dog? What will happen to it when everyone is out at work? What are the alternatives?" Or she would ask who was going to clean the stairs, how often people felt they should be cleaned and in what way. The decisions were made by the group. That is important.'

In the early days, some of the residents were over-excited and tired themselves out. One young woman allowed the freedom to go to her head and refused to go to work (some residents had outside jobs, some attended a centre). She got no sympathy from the others and had to return to the hostel – and pay off her rent arrears!

Supervision at The Cherries amounted to one half-time social worker, one domestic two mornings a week, briefed to keep an eye open for problems, a rent collector calling once a week and a social worker not connected with the scheme, but who lived nearby and could pop in some evenings to say hello. Nobody, once the initial nucleus was established, lived in.

When they are not working, the residents can go out – swimming in a group, to the pub, to the cinema, shopping – or stay in to watch television, play darts or table tennis. They can also of course, do nothing. There are no organized activities. They still keep contact with the hostel, some people opting to go on holiday with the hostel group.

CONCLUSIONS

Those involved with The Cherries set out to prove (a) that Group Homes were the cheapest way of housing the mentally handicapped (they felt it was pretty generally accepted as the best) and (b) that people with IQ levels previously considered impossible could live in this way. They proved the first beyond doubt. Many people believe they proved the second too – but possibly they just proved that IQ tests are unreliable.

Many local mentally handicapped societies all over the country are currently planning or running their own Group Homes, but a lot of parents still remain unconvinced that their child would be capable of living unsupervised.

The secret of success must, I think, remain flexibility. There is room for a variety of homes, with varying degrees of supervision. One small society has rented a council house on behalf of four mentally handicapped people, next door to a dedicated member of the society who spends several evenings and weekends with them. She has involved her grown-up family and several neighbours, so the residents have a lot of support. They could not, she believes, survive unsupervised, with only a social worker calling twice a week.

You have, as the social worker said, to play it by ear. But it has to be a sensitive ear, to listen out for signs of strain, of disharmony – which could, for the wrong mentally handicapped person, be much greater than in any supervised, untrendy home or hostel.

*Two annual reports on life at The Cherries were produced by D. G. and D. M. Race. See p. 205 for details.

4

Voluntary Agencies – Still Filling the Gaps

You would think we would not need them – all these homes and communities being set up by parents' groups and voluntary organizations. You would think that by now the Welfare State would have found all the gaps and covered them with their much-lauded net.

Far from it. Instead of diminishing, voluntary provision for the mentally handicapped is on the increase, a positive growth industry. Parents are partly responsible. They believe in voluntary agencies, in charitable groups working from the heart, not the head, and definitely not from the wallet.

Only the scene has changed. The voluntary sector is no longer in the hands of gentle Christian souls but efficient professionals, who know how to balance the books and woo donations from multinational corporations. Far more rewarding than the collecting tin. Charities have become big business and can be as competitive and cut-throat as any other business.

Neither is it all run on charity. The bill for most children and adults in private Homes is paid by their Local Authority and state allowances. This way, basic living costs are covered and donations go towards capital building projects and the little extras that make life more pleasant. The biggest fund-raising efforts tend to go towards getting the places started. Strict Local Authority regulations concerning such points as fire precautions and the number of washbasins can make this prohibitively expensive to small groups.

Many of the successful Homes were started by parents but few are actually run by them. They have handed over to the Local Authority or installed administrators, matrons and managers. I feel that those where parents remain actively involved and have a say in policy are the best – for parents and their children, anyway. Staff do not always see the advantages.

The niggling worry about the older, more insular establishments is how little control there may be on standards of care. True, each home has to be registered and there are minimum standards laid down, but enforcing them is not always practicable. It would, you feel, take a major outcry to have one closed down and the residents made homeless. As one manager pointed out, he is always forewarned about inspectors' visits – which makes it a fairly pointless exercise if he has anything to hide.

These small homes, and even some of the large ones, are in effect governed by one person's beliefs – be they good, bad or indifferent. It makes them very vulnerable to bad practice and bad management.

But that's the bad news. At best, they have the freedom to be experimental in the best way without getting tied up in red tape like the statutory Homes. In general they are not so imaginative in their concepts of care as they might be, tending to stick to traditional paths. In fact, you can brush the cobwebs off some of the ideas and practices prevalent in a few of the small Homes.

Where, for instance, are the small units catering for the severely multiply handicapped or including them among their abler residents? Practically non-existent, yet here is a desperate need and one some of the voluntary organizations could, with a little imagination and effort, fill.

Harry Neal, Secretary of the recently formed Association of Residential Communities for the Retarded (ARC) is aware of this gap in provision. ARC is a union of the most respected organizations providing residential care. It exists to keep an eye on standards, to advise new groups entering the field who may find it confusing and, by banding together, to give the voluntary sector some muscle as a group.

Mr Neal, who also works for the National Society for Mentally Handicapped Children,* is keen to see an increase in voluntary places for the severely handicapped of all ages – not only those with multiple handicaps but what he calls 'the fifty per cent of all mentally handicapped who are non-contributors, the people who are largely ignored by groups starting Homes'.

He believes strongly in villages and sheltered communities and would like to see the established, successful places agreeing to take a proportion of non-contributors.

The National Society, too, is 'committed to the idea of village-type care for the severely handicapped'. It is a glimmer of hope,

*The National Society for Mentally Handicapped Children produces a useful book listing statutory and non-statutory units: *Directory of Residential Accommodation for the Mentally Handicapped in England and Wales*.

though it is obvious that 'villages' filled with highly dependent people would have to be different in many ways from those we know now. Different to the point of being totally unrecognizable and possibly more like hospitals with small units and a non-medical bias.

Round the circle goes again. But at least thoughts in the voluntary sector are at last being turned towards the greatest gap of all.

Provision for Children

WESTRIDGE – COMBINING SCHOOL AND HOME

I went to Westridge with a preconceived idea. This couldn't be helped. I had heard a lot about this Children's Home – a few cynical remarks, but mostly glowing praise.

Local parents see it as the Eton or Harrow of the mentally handicapped world, the place you automatically nominate first choice if you think of finding a residential place for your child. And, as around fifty applicants are turned down for every one accepted, the place you rarely get.

One mother, a little more cynical or perhaps realistic, than most, wonders if she is the only parent ever to have turned down the offer of a place for her son. She was shown round on a warm, summer day, she says, and was immediately put off by the fact that all the children were sitting in their bedrooms.

'I got the feeling it was a place for the wealthy to put their children away in the nicest possible way.'

Feature writers in newspapers and magazines have waxed quite lyrical, bearing in mind that reporters with no specialist knowledge and a page to fill are not necessarily totally objective witnesses.

('You feel the children are growing, however painfully, like flowers towards the light . . . .' . . . 'You leave with your pity for the children transformed into admiration. They do experience some of the richness of human life . . .' The staff are described as having 'a degree of dedication most of us are incapable of, and the sort of love we can hardly begin to understand'.)

More down-to-earth are remarks from professionals who work with the mentally handicapped and know Westridge and its children.

'Every child who leaves there has Westridge stamped on him. You would never mistake it. It makes them polite and well-behaved and they find it very hard to fit into the rougher places they have to go to at sixteen.'

'It's a lovely place, but they're a bit cranky.'

'It's beautiful outside, but they spend more on the gardens than on the buildings and staffing.'

So what do you make of all this when you have never seen the place? I imagined a remote eighteenth-century building, staffed by ethereal beings of great dedication but little modern knowledge; filled mainly with the children of parents wealthy enough to pay the fees. And most of all, full of 'easy option' children. Knowing so many people who had been turned away, I'd assumed they took only the more able, educable children.

A lot of preconceived notions – both good and bad – bit the dust. Westridge has changed radically over the past decade and outgrown the myths that sprang up around it in its early days. Today it has to function as a school which will satisfy education inspectors (which meant compromising on its old 'spiritual' methods) and as a Home, which is struggling now to comply with new, higher Local Authority standards. It is not the place it was, the place most parents still believe it is. Whether that is good or bad depends on your point of view.

Westridge lies at the foot of gently rolling hills, up a long drive, off country roads. There are sheep grazing, daffodils blooming, trees and shrubs doing their own thing in landscaped profusion and – nearer the Victorian mansion itself – the steady buzz of lawn-mowers.

Not a sight or sound of the motorways, though they are not far off these days. Westridge, in its fifty acres of parkland, was isolated from the world, when it opened its doors to the handicapped in 1932 – but the world has crept up on it.

The house is still the heart of the place, with its big hall, where all 110 children meet for Morning-song, the dining-room that has been doubled in size and the decidedly un-Victorian kitchens with their own bakery, where all the cooking is done. New buildings have been tacked around the periphery – in particular an up-to-date school, where all the children, except a few of the very youngest, attend morning and afternoon sessions. In theory, Westridge takes children from babyhood to sixteen, but the youngest at the moment are four-year-olds. The oldest – a middle-aged man who for some reason never moved on and now has a room to himself and helps around the Home.

There is also a young man, who cannot be placed elsewhere because of a serious heart condition and whose parents made financial arrangements years ago for him to be looked after for life. He has his own room, with unbreakable wired glass and a door that cannot be opened from the inside. 'He smashes things up,' said a staff member, explaining the windows. 'Unfortunately he smashes up small children, too.' He indicated the locked door.

From my point of view, trying to represent each category of residential establishment, the interesting point about Westridge is that it is a Home with its own boarding-school. The children live and attend school in the same group of buildings, not going out to Local Authority schools like their counterparts in most modern Homes. It narrows their horizons.

But in a general way, the main difference between Westridge and the other places in the book is that it is a Steiner Home, based on the fairly individual Christian principles of the Austrian philosopher Rudolph Steiner, who died in 1925.

Without getting too involved, this encompasses a belief in reincarnation. To quote their own literature: 'The causes of mental handicap must be sought partly in a previous existence and some of the help given today will only bear fruit in the far future.' One mother I know with two mentally handicapped children remembers the shock of being told there that this was punishment for bad behaviour in a previous existence. Nevertheless she thought the Home 'wonderful'. Steiner called the mentally handicapped (though little of his writing was directly concerned with them) 'children in need of special care of the soul'.

However you feel about all this, the end-product was a collection of people with strong Christian principles and a deep love of the children in their charge. Westridge in the early days was a close, dedicated community, made up of resident workers from all backgrounds who turned their hand to any job with missionary zeal, took no wages and claimed only necessary expenses from a communal fund.

The most unusual custom as far as they affected the children and their families was the practice of insisting that all residents stay put over the high points of the year – Christmas and Easter. The festivals were celebrated as a group in the Home.

This no longer happens. Children who can go home for Easter and Christmas do so – and for summer holidays if possible, to relieve pressure on the staff when there is no school. It came about, Mr B – one of the directors – explained, because staff were no longer prepared to work at holiday times. They wanted to be with their own families.

Mr B has been involved with Westridge for twenty-five years, mainly dealing with administrative work. His wife, a dauntingly hard-working lady, is Matron. They live nearby with their children, the youngest of whom is now a teenager, but Mrs B often does not go off-duty until 10 p.m. after a full day's work, and sometimes stays overnight.

Though they were among the pioneers, they are both forward-thinking and happy to welcome changes for the better. There were some big changes in 1971, following the 1970 Education Act. The children had always received education but on the lines laid down by the directors, with teachers qualified only in Steiner methods and taught by older, experienced colleagues.

When schools for the mentally handicapped came under the jurisdiction of the Education Authorities, in order to be officially recognized as a boarding-school, Westridge had to bring in its quota of qualified teachers. Most were young women – there are very few men at Westridge – with modern methods, who had not heard of the name Steiner.

'We were probably complacent,' Mr B says. 'We had to change and we achieved new levels of efficiency.'

Mrs B agrees. 'You have to change with the times. You cannot ignore the outside world. It has a lot to offer. I would rather see staff who are not interested in Rudolph Steiner but are interested in mentally handicapped children, than the other way round – which you sometimes got in the past. I would like to combine the old caring attitude with the new methods as they come along.'

There are 126 staff directly involved with the children. Of these, ten come in daily; the others are resident. Nobody is coy about wages. Teachers earn £30 a week; the daily nursing assistants £24; 'students', with some qualification like NNEB, earn £18; and completely unqualified students (often girls filling in six months or a year before going on to university or full-time training) get £10.

'We keep our fees low by under-paying our staff,' said Mrs B, who is inclined to be alarmingly blunt at times. ('Must you? Couldn't you go somewhere else?' she said, when I asked to spend some time at Westridge – then, when I turned up, offered me freedom to come and go as I pleased.) Mrs B does not feel resident staff are badly done by, 'although I know some of the young girls do. Their board and lodging makes up a lot of the difference'.

The ill wind of unemployment has blown some good in the direction of places like Westridge. There is no shortage of teachers or nursing help. They rely heavily on teenage girls, but most of them now have some qualification, usually nursery nursing. In the past the bulk of the help was still young people, but from overseas and Steiner-orientated, using the Home as the practical part of a training course.

Westridge is a limited company, run by directors appointed by the trustees. Fees are, at the time of writing, £2,992 a year, with all but twelve children paid for jointly by their Local Education Department and the Social Services. Another myth wiped out – that the children are from wealthy families. At one time, the bulk of children were paid for privately, but now most are referred by social workers and many come from very poor backgrounds. Of the twelve who are fee-paying, eleven are from overseas.

It is a charity, and heavily subsidized by fund-raising, much of it organized by a local woman who acts as a highly efficient public relations officer.

Thursday 10.30 a.m. The classroom

In Nora's class, seven of the youngest children are at morning school in one of the new, bright classrooms. The only visible difference from any nursery class is a religious picture on the wall. A couple of them are looking through picture books with a young helper; two are shuffling around on their bottoms on the floor (Westridge does not take physically handicapped children, except those that show promise of walking; some simply don't keep the promise). Andy and Joss, six-year-old mongols and inseparable friends, are sitting in the window and another non-walker, a little boy from the Middle East, is flashing stunning smiles and fluttering long eyelashes.

A couple of days later, on another visit, I meet the same child sitting in a pushchair that is held together by optimism and string, being readied for a train trip to London to see his father, with one of the young helpers. She looked very young for the responsibility of a long trip with a handicapped child. The helpers are given a lot of responsibility and freedom at Westridge. The red tape is rarely visible.

Nora came to Westridge soon after it opened. Her husband works there, too. To put her two children through a normal Steiner school, at a time when staff were paid no wages, she worked in the kitchens. She never qualified as a teacher in the conventional sense and is scornful of modern methods.

'Behaviour modification! All this jargon they use – I can't remember half of it. You find out it means something very simple. The latest idea is rewarding them for good behaviour, isn't it? Like training a dog. They try to teach intellectually now and ignore the whole child. You can help these children to improve, but you cannot change them into something they are not. You cannot make them what we call normal. Why try? They can teach us so much the way they are.'

To the children she sings instruction and information in little rhymes. She teaches them, she says, mainly by example. They will hopefully copy her words and actions and social skills. This last term she interprets as good manners, not the way it is used by modern educationalists. There is no doubt of her sincerity or kindness, but it is strange to go into a classroom where the teacher is not working to a set programme of some kind for each child, at least in theory, even if she does not get the time to put it into practice.

It happens, I am told, in most other classes in the school, with older children and young qualified teachers. 'I think the inspectors would like to see all our older teachers gone and replaced by younger ones,' Mrs B told me one day.

Just before 12.15 p.m. the children sit in a circle on little chairs and Nora reads them a story, a familiar story punctuated with plenty of animal noises, with which they are expected to join in. Only Joss and Andy do. They are more able than most of the others and together they are very self-sufficient and as naughty as any normal six-year-olds. The two dark-haired, non-ambulant little boys from overseas just want to communicate with smiles and looks. When Nora gets to the bit about the 'poor little bunny rabbit' and strokes each child's head, they love it.

'Quiet as mice,' Nora tells them, 'the mummy mice are waiting outside.' The door opens on a group of girls, who scoop up the children to take them back to their respective 'nurseries' for tidying up before lunch.

12.15 p.m. – Nursery 1

The residential areas of Westridge are divided into 'nurseries' – each one a dormitory, with its own toilets and bathroom nearby. These also function as playrooms – hence one parent's complaint that the children were in their bedrooms in the afternoons. There are no separate 'living rooms'. Each unit is fairly autonomous, run by the people who work there – the same group all the time, except for staff changes. They look after their charges, give them their meals, put them to bed, take them to school, take them out when they can.

It sounds nice, but can lead occasionally to a lack of supervision. 'There ought to be more spot checks on the nurseries,' one of the staff told me. 'I wouldn't trust some of the girls here, to look after a cat, and they get far too much freedom. They run their nursery as they want to. One girl took some children out one weekend and left a girl locked in the backroom. For safety, she said. The child turned the taps on and flooded the room when she got bored. Just imagine what could have happened.'

Not all the children in Nora's class are in the same nursery. Only three of the boys – Joss, Andy and Alex, who is a wheelchair case – go up to the same unit.

Here they join three other boys – as in many residential places, boys greatly outnumber girls – Jonathan, Richard, an engaging four-year-old Down's Syndrome boy, and nine-year-old David, the oldest in the group.

Jonathan and David are brain-damaged and sometimes difficult to handle. Alex is severely handicapped. The three mongol children, far more sociable and capable, help to balance them, and the nurseries are arranged with this in mind.

Mrs B told me: 'I wouldn't have a mongol in the place if it was up to me. I prefer to take the more difficult brain-damaged children – the ones nobody wants. Mongols fit in anywhere. Still, I suppose they give a sense of balance to the place.'

She says she also aims to take the majority of their children from the lowest IQ range: below 40 – another surprise to me – but refuses physically handicapped children 'because it would not be fair to expect the young girls to lift them'. Not quite a valid reason, I felt, with children only up to sixteen, and the girls looking energetic enough.

But they would take more staff and create problems, undoubtedly. Mrs B chooses children for the few places available, she says, on the basis of who can be helped most at Westridge. It is her decision with another director and a doctor.

The nursery is in the charge of two students and two day helpers. Liz, the unqualified student, is away today, her weekly day off. Janet, the second student, is energetic, brisk and unemotional with the children and slightly rebellious ('I don't like being called a student. I'm not – I'm a trained nursery nurse'). She works split shifts: 7 to 9.30 a.m. to get the children out of bed, breakfasted and into school; 12.10 to 2.00 p.m. to cover lunch, and 4 to 8.00 p.m., from school till bedtime.

Lynn is a day girl, straight from school, working from 7 to 3.00 p.m. Denise, the oldest and the only married woman, with a five-year-old daughter, works from 9 till 3.00 p.m.

Nobody is officially in charge, they explain, but somehow Denise seems to be. She tends to suggest what should be done, often speaks for the nursery as a whole and is fast and efficient in dealing with the children. Still in her twenties, she has long blonde hair and long painted nails. She looks frivolous, glamorous and absolutely wrong for the job, but turns out to be friendly, natural and totally right for it.

Mrs B says: 'I like to have a slightly older woman in each nursery, with a stable background and experience of children. They can usually be sharp with the young girls if need be – and some of them do need it.'

The children go straight from school to the bathroom. David has a convulsion and is dealt with routinely by Janet, whilst the others carry on with the washing and the toileting.

It is a small room, with a bath, a changing area, a wash-basin and two toilets divided by partitions. The partitions are recent additions, part of the changes suggested by Local Authority inspectors to bring the residential area of the Home up to scratch.

Westridge is currently facing criticism from these quarters and trying hard to conform. In theory, because they are below official requirements, they could have their licence as a mental nursing home revoked and be closed down. The likelihood of this happening, though, is remote. What would the various Local Authorities do if the children were left on their hands?

Westridge staff tend to regard the demands as impractical and over-zealous. The logic of removing locks from the nursery doors so high that children could not reach them was accepted. Children being trapped in a fire was considered a greater danger than their running away. But other suggestions, like a 'home place' for each child, a personal wardrobe and locker by each bed, is deemed ridiculous.

'They do not realize the sort of children we have here,' explained one staff member. If they could reach cupboards, they would pull everything out of them. Having their own locker does not mean a thing to a lot of them.' The large clothes cupboards – one for each nursery, big enough to hold each child's clothes – stay out in the hallways.

Other innovations forced on them by the Local Authority, such as the partitions between the toilets, for privacy, are also unpopular.

'The children, particularly the young ones, do not want privacy,' Denise pointed out. 'They are not inhibited. Why try to make them so? Two or three of them go into the toilet together anyway, despite the partitions. In a bathroom as small as this, anything extra is unwelcome. It leaves hardly any space to stand while you bath them.'

12.30 p.m.

Along the corridors, down narrow steps, across a big hall, to the dining-room with its big, scrubbed tables. It is very clean, almost spartan. Two children are carried, the rest walk. All the children in Westridge are accommodated at one sitting, each nursery to its own table and their staff eating with them.

Two of the girls disappear behind the counter that separates the kitchen from the dining-room and return with the children's meals – a mixture of chopped chicken, vegetables and potato. The adults queue for self-service – chicken curry or a vegetarian meal. There are a lot of vegetarians on the staff.

Before a bit is eaten, staff and children, all those who are able, join hands and chant: 'Blessings on the meal'.

All the children, except Alex, can feed themselves – mostly with spoons and with varying degrees of competence. Denise sits beside Alex, lightly holds his nose till he opens his mouth, then pops in a spoonful of the mashed mixture. There is a fair amount of self-generated mess around. Andy holds out his hand to be wiped, but there is not a tissue or cloth in sight. The mess has to be borne.

David, who can feed himself, but prefers not to, shoves his plate towards the nearest adult. It is shoved back and he is told to get on with it.

The staff ratio is impressive, three to six, but it does not always work out. 'Sometimes we are falling over each other,' Janet says. 'At other times there will be just one person on. It is worst at weekends, with Denise and Lynn not in.'

'Sometimes there is only one on and, with two wheelchair cases, you can't take the children out all day. In good weather, if there are two of us, we take them around the fields for a walk.'

There is rice pudding for after, then more holding of hands and a chant of: 'Thank you and goodbye'. Back to the bathroom. More toileting, face wiping and teeth cleaning (each child has his own mug, cloth and toothbrush). Those who are able gulp down the water out of their tooth mugs, those who cannot are not offered any. They were not given a drink before, during or after their meal. Incredibly, they do not get one at midday – only at breakfast and tea and with biscuits after school.

They are back to school for 2 p.m. Janet and Lynn take them. It is Denise's afternoon at the pool. Westridge boasts a hydro-therapy pool, a dark, silent place, the only lights under the water. Taking the physically handicapped children down here for treatment and helping them in the water is one of Denise's 'odd jobs'. Another is taking the children for hair-cutting when a hairdresser comes in.

She loves working with the children, but coming in as she does during school hours, she only sees them at lunch-time. She calls herself 'housemother', though it is not an official staff title at Westridge, and defines her job as 'being a substitute mother to the children in my nursery'.

At the moment, though, only Richard is at home with her in the nursery during the day and Denise complains of feeling like a glorified cleaner, with housework her main task. The next time I see her she has approached Mrs B with her problem and a new deal has been worked out – Denise will come in on Saturdays instead of Fridays, to spend at least one full day with the children. Fortunately the system is flexible.

Monday 10.00 a.m.

Denise is downstairs in the big hall having coffee with a few more staff members. A group of visitors have been shown round and are leaving. There are not many visiting parties these days. There used to be a steady stream, which tended to interrupt the work, so they had to cut down on them.

When the visitors do come, mostly on Sundays, they get a fairly organized tour – perhaps taking in a group of children doing a play in the small hall. (There is also a large, modern hall which doubles for the regular Sunday services attended by all.) Invariably guests see the new gymnasium in the school and the pool.

Denise takes me up to the nursery, where she has left Richard playing on his own on the floor. He is responsive and attractive. In the dining-room, staff members often come up to play with him and give him a cuddle. Like all babies, he gets the lion's share of attention.

He and the other two little mongols get taken out and taken home for weekends by the girls on the nursery. The staff are encouraged to take the children out. Denise is very aware that the more endearing trio get all the perks and says she tries to give the other three extra playtime and attention to make up for it. Nevertheless, it was Andy she had home for Christmas.

On the previous Friday, Richard's grandparents had visited him. Denise was delighted to get the opportunity to meet them and assure them he was happy. They were, she felt, very satisfied with the situation. 'And I was so glad I'd stuck the postcards they sent him on the wall. At least they could see we take an interest and do not throw them away.'

All the girls said they would love to meet parents, but rarely got the chance and only know little snippets of information about the family and background. Occasionally there is an unexpected contact. Andy's family live in America. A girl who used to help look after him there before he came to the Home recently sent him a postcard and Denise wrote back a long letter about his progress. The ex-nannie now plans a trip to visit Andy, staying at Denise's home.

The nursery is old-fashioned and high-ceilinged, with 'institutional green' gloss paint on the walls and brown vinyl tiles on the floor. Decidedly spartan, but the girls have stuck up transfers, photographs, cards and mobiles and there are toys, big and small, around the room.

Each nursery is precisely what the people in charge of it make it. It is theirs to make or mar. The day housemother, in particular, is in charge of cleaning, tidying and decorating it.

The first one I had seen was a completely bare shell of a room, with a broken window, scribble on the walls and five bare beds lining the walls around an empty expanse of floor.

Denise's nursery, on the other hand, is homely and spotlessly clean. She treats it, she says, as if it were her own home, even to bringing in unwanted toys. During school holidays, her five-year-old daughter comes in.

Denise came to Westridge after working in an office and fostering normal children, for a notoriously sentimental reason . . . that 'it could have been my child'. There had been concern that her daughter might have suffered brain damage at birth. After two years she has perfected the art of combining sentimentality with a practical talent for home-making.

Richard is wearing white cotton mittens. If he doesn't, he scratches his ears till they are raw. Nobody seems to have worked out why he does this, but Denise made the mittens, as prevention if not cure. 'They wanted to put him in restraining harness at night. I'd hate that.'

Richard sits on her lap, hiding his face and peeping. He is one of the most settled, un-neurotic children I have seen in care. Denise has looked after him since he arrived, less than a year ago, so he has had the stability of a constant mother-substitute and virtually a one-to-one relationship. Whether he will still be as happy when he is at school and only seeing her at lunch-time, I could not guess.

Denise's morning is spent like any housewife at home – cleaning, tidying, fetching clothes from the laundry, labelling them if necessary, mending. The large cupboard in the hall holds all items of clothing – supplied by parents where they keep in touch, bought by the Home if they do not.

It is amazingly tidy, each garment buttoned and folded as though straight from a top-class laundry, though they will only be worn once. Denise does all this, though there is no rule about it. She is just, she says, inclined to be houseproud and tidy – a fact which no doubt irritates some of her co-workers.

'You have to have your standards and mine don't change when I come here. I do everything as I would at home. This is home to these children. If you open a cupboard in some of the other nurseries, a pile of messy clothes will fall out on your head.'

What happens when other helpers do not aspire to such standards? 'I have no power to make them do it my way, but I mention how we do things here. We had a girl once who insisted on trying to toilet-train Jonathan. A waste of time. The poor kid has a hard enough life as I see it. Why put him through that as well? He cannot understand.

'Now with Richard, I am toilet-training him and I'll give him a smack if he does something wrong. He understands, you see. I hate to see children who don't understand get smacked.

'One of the girls here sits with her elbows on the table at meals and then smacks Andy when he does the same. I hit her with the ladle when I saw her doing it the other day, just playfully, but I think she sees the sense now. If I caught someone doing something I really disapproved of, I would have to mention it to Mrs B. She misses very little, actually.'

The care assistants get no training. They are placed where there is a vacancy but can be moved to another nursery if they are unhappy there. Occasional personality clashes necessitate this. 'Sometimes they are more trouble to me than the children,' said Mrs B wryly.

Their knowledge of mental handicap is sadly lacking. Was Alex microcephalic, I wondered, and received some blank looks. 'We used to be able to look at the children's notes if we wanted to,' one girl said, 'but I don't think we can now'. Perhaps it helps them to see the children as individuals, less as cases. But still, I can't see how a little learning could be a bad thing.

In this nursery, at least, they are not working to any set goals or on any organized programme with the children. A tremendous amount of faith is placed in the commonsense of the care staff, given that their practical experience, has often only been with normal children.

I am all for democracy, but in this setting it must be confusing. Surely someone should be in charge of each nursery and have the final say in how things are done?

'We work as a team,' one of them insisted, but admits that there are woolly areas which cause friction. If a morning group do the absolute minimum, only getting the children ready and leaving a dirty bathroom for the next person who comes on duty, there is bound to be bad feeling. There are no rules to say which job belongs to whom and fair play is not necessarily a part of everyone's make-up. It is, presumably, a hangover from the old days when all work was accepted and shared for spiritual reward only.

Things change. Few of the students stay long. 'Six months is about the average,' one of them told me. 'There is no point, especially if you have done some training. All you get is experience. There is no chance of a career. What can you be promoted to?'

Some do stay, of course – or used to. Mrs B began as a lowly, unqualified helper. She has no doubt there will be others happy to replace her. 'You will always find people prepared to do a job as rewarding as this, however demanding,' she said.

Wednesday 6.00 p.m.

The children from the nursery are in the dining-room. Liz, the unqualified student, is with them, alone. (It is Janet's day off.) She is an intelligent, polite girl from a medical family, filling in time before she starts training as a nurse. Looking for something to do meanwhile, not necessarily with the mentally handicapped, she found the job advertised in *The Lady*.

Like most of the students, her home is in another part of the country, so she lives in. It is a very quiet life, she says. No social outlets except for the pub. She does a lot of knitting.

The children are in their pyjamas and dressing-gowns. Since school ended, she has bathed all of them, single-handed, leaving the others in the nursery. Getting them down to the dining-room, with two who have to be carried, has not been easy; neither is trying to see they all get some food and do not run around and make a nuisance of themselves, as Andy and Joss do when bored.

Liz is up and down constantly, supervising and feeding, leaving no time to eat her own small salad. She is new to that nursery, she explains (though she has been at Westridge for six months) and does not know the children and their foibles very well yet.

Alex refuses his scrambled egg and tomato mixture and she does not force him. Andy spends his time trying to join the children at the next table. David keeps taking off his slippers. Joss gets down and turns his chair upside down. Jonathan falls asleep and Richard, after testing a spoonful, hurls his plate across the table with an expression of disgust.

It is becoming very like the Mad Hatter's tea party – Liz aware of her inability to cope single-handed and me aware she would do a lot better if she were not self-conscious about my being there. She is concerned about Richard: 'He doesn't eat egg, I remember now. What would he eat?'

She goes away and comes back with a yoghourt, a regular standby. Richard spoons up every last drop and looks hopefully into the empty carton. It does not seem a big tea. There is a small piece of bread and cheese each afterwards, but only a few of them want it. Richard doesn't like cheese either.

There is orange squash in a big jug to drink and they are all, not surprisingly, thirsty and eager for that. Richard pushes back his cup for second, third, fourth helpings. Liz wonders about giving him too much. Alex, unable to ask, only gets one small beaker-full.

Some of the other tables have bread and jam on them, but not this one. Apparently it is left to the staff to get it if their children like it, and these don't. None of them has eaten a substantial amount. It would be difficult for one person to see that they did or even notice that they had not.

Before we go back upstairs, a fraught-looking Liz stops to have a word with Mrs B. She is given a highly efficient helper, a woman who normally deals with laundry. From then on, the going is easy, with the two women working together.

In the bathroom, all children who need them are put into towelling nappies. No plastic pants. One of the impractical rules of the house is that no child wears these protective garments over nappies. It explains at last the number of wet bottoms in the classroom.

'They restrict movement and leave marks on the legs,' one staff member explained. Wet clothing and bedding is even more uncomfortable, I would imagine.

Did she usually get extra help on the day she is alone, I asked Liz. No, she didn't. How did she cope? 'Slowly but surely,' she laughed.

By 7.30 p.m. all six children are in bed, but they get out again regularly and have to be persuaded back. The bottom sheets are not fitted and the coverings are not duvets but blankets and bedspreads, so it all slides off and within minutes there are apple-pie beds all round.

The children have been reluctant to go to sleep since the long evenings began. The curtains, hung between the glass and wire grating, cannot be closed because someone lost the key. Janet can operate them with a surgical appliance, but nobody else dares risk breaking it.

David keeps taking off his nappy and throwing the clothes off. Liz sits on the end of his bed and reads a story. Andy and Joss listen, the others ignore her. It is nearly time for her to go off duty. At eight, night staff come on. One woman who uses the dispensary as her base keeps an eye on a group of nurseries. Dispensary is a bit of a misnomer. There is no registered nurse at Westridge, which is a sore point with Local Authority inspectors.

It has never caused any problems. A doctor who lives nearby is readily available and the children, the staff point out, are no more likely to be ill than their normal peers.

The itinerary is different in other nurseries with older children. After school, they are usually taken outside to play – there is a well-equipped-play area – or for a walk. Bath time for them will be after tea.

'At one time,' one of the staff told me, 'they used to bath the children, whatever their ages, immediately after school, so there would not be so much to do after tea and they could finish nice and early. But that has been stopped. It meant that the children were ready for bed just after school.'

Each nursery has books, toys, games and writing equipment – playthings matched to the ages and abilities of the children who live there. The old puritanical tradition still forbids television. There is not a set in the place. 'Though I sometimes think we should have one for the older children,' Mr B said, half-serious, 'to break them in and get them used to it for when they leave here.'

Entertainment instead centres around eurythmy and music at weekends and evenings for older children. There are plays put on by the children – even the nursery joins in this. 'Our Joss was a black sheep in one,' said Denise, 'type-casting, we all said.'

Easter and Christmas and the weeks leading up to the festivals are still celebrated in great spiritual style and all the children attend Sunday service in the big hall. Each summer there is a seaside holiday for all the children.

Conclusions

Even if it is not Utopia, Westridge has more going for it than many Homes of a similar size. But it suffers from one unavoidable drawback: it caters for children up to the age of sixteen only. What then? A few children go on to adult Homes based on the same principles, but these have a static population, so there are not nearly enough vacancies to go round. Others go to hostels in the community – and what a shock that must be after the sheltered atmosphere of the Home.

Nothing in Westridge prepares them for going out by day to a training centre and by night to a club – or for travelling around by bus and getting to know a wide variety of neighbours. One older staff member talked worriedly of seeing ex-residents turn into 'regular pub crawlers' because there was no discipline and no carefully-chosen entertainment on the premises to keep them occupied.

A few – very few, the staff insist – can only be accommodated in mental handicap hospitals. Wherever they go, most will be ill-prepared for the outside world.

In a general way, Westridge top brass tends to disapprove of the current trend encouraging parents to keep their children at home. It is not, they say, realistic or fair to the rest of the family. Mr B believes that social workers are brain-washed into seeing family care as the ideal, with no experience of the reality and the problems.

That said, Westridge cannot hope to provide a much larger slice of the care it advocates, in the near future. It has grown – too much, some of the older staff think – and is still growing, but more slowly.

It is still a self-contained, fairly isolated community – just the sort of place the integrationalists would stamp out. All the time, though, it gets more forward-looking and more outgoing. More – dare one say it? – ordinary. It is inevitable. Going two ways at once becomes rather uncomfortable, and forward is the obvious direction. It would be a pity, though, if it has to sacrifice all of its unique, old-fashioned caring to progress.

NO. 5, THE AVENUE – MULTIPLY HANDICAPPED CHILDREN

This is one of the few small Homes taking multiply handicapped children. Small is relative – there are twenty-four children living there, about half considered too handicapped to be acceptable at local Special Schools, where there is a shortage of special care places.

A Development Unit, which is actually an on-the-spot special care class, funded by the Local Authority and staffed by a teacher and two assistants, was set up in the grounds six years ago. But there is a group of children considered too severely handicapped even to attend this – though that is a matter for some debate – and these are ones I was most interested in.

Number 5 was once a private house, overlooking a suburban green with a nice village feel, three miles out of a northern city. It is private, opened in 1964 by a charitable organization. The matron, a brisk no-nonsense lady in blue uniform, who has been there eleven years, makes financing sound like a matter of keeping your fingers crossed and offering an occasional prayer.

'We've no capital behind us. We are dependent on voluntary help – good friends, benevolent funds and local firms.' Donations listed in her ledger vary from £2 to £350 from a car factory.

In fact the Local Authorities are the biggest contributors, paying the basic £52-a-week fee for each child. This is, relatively speaking, very low, particularly considering the dependency of the children. It doesn't leave much over for treats. Parents – those who have not lost contact – contribute when and if they can. Often is it just the occasional £5 or £1 note sent in.

Staffing, in the senior ranks, is impressive: Matron, her deputy, three SRNs (part-time), two SENs, one RMN, one NNEB and eight young nursery assistants, who do most of the washing, changing and feeding. They need trained staff on duty, Matron says, because of the number of children 'physically at risk'. Mostly because of their fits, she means.

Allowing for shifts, holidays and illness, it is still a high staff ratio. All the more shattering, then, to find five profoundly handicapped children lying all day, every day, in a pleasant but crowded room called the Nursery and one little spastic girl alone in a gloomy room next door, staring at the ceiling from her iron cot, with nothing to do. They are fed, dressed, changed, washed in their cots.

These children do not attend the Development Unit (except for one six-year-old girl who had been over for a couple of hours). Why? The practical reason is that the unit is full up. Mrs R, the teacher, can only take nine children and until she can move one on to a day school outside, there is not much she can do. She is, however, very much aware and concerned for this group of children who have lain for years, day in, day out, unstimulated, in the nursery. She seems to be the only one who is.

But the nursery children were never suggested as pupils anyway. Because, the senior staff point out, these children are cot cases. They are not well. They have fits. They will never walk or feed themselves. They will always be in nappies, so what is the point of getting them out of their cots? This is the way it has always been.

A similar situation existed in the hospital ward where six profoundly handicapped teenagers lived, but the winds of change had blown more strongly through the hospital. The staff were aware that it was less than ideal. Some of them at least were far from complacent and wanted to see changes.

Here, it did not seem to have occurred to anyone that there might be something lacking in the lives of the children in the Nursery. Except to the teacher, who was in no position to change it and anyway had come in from outside, so to speak. The nursery assistants, sixteen-to-eighteen-year-olds filling in time before going on to a 'proper' job or dabbling their toes tentatively to see if they might fancy this kind of work, simply accepted it. They knew nothing different, after all.

Of four I talked to, one had just started that week, two had been there a couple of months. The fourth, an energetic, forthright girl who had, amazingly, been there three years, launched into a diatribe about how they rarely took even the abler children out locally because the neighbours didn't like it, before she was whisked away.

One change from the old days: a physiotherapist comes into the Nursery twice a week to do exercises with the children. Doesn't he give the girls some simple exercises to do with them on the other days? They have, after all, plenty of free time when the children are at school.

Gasps of horror. They couldn't do what a physiotherapist does. They might harm the children. Agreement from the trained nurse, who has been working at the Home since it opened. Besides, they are quite busy with nappy changes and feeding.

Do they play with them? Surprise. Not with the Nursery children – but they do play with the others when they come in from school.

One of the senior staff said that she doesn't leave the young girls too long on duty in the Nursery because it is 'depressing' for them, 'really soul-destroying'. It must be even more so when they are given nothing constructive to do and never taught to see the children as individuals rather than bottoms to wash and faces to feed.

Thursday 12 noon

The children from the Development Unit have been taken across the yard to the dining-room, where the Nursery assistants feed them or help those who can manage a little. A few of the children have additional physical handicaps. All are highly dependent.

The teacher, Mrs R, would prefer to organize lunch at school – basically one large room with the necessary offices opening off it – so that it could be part of the training programme. But that was not generally acceptable. So the teaching staff bring in biscuits and provide drinks so that the children can have feeding practice at school.

One little girl, for instance, cannot chew at all, the part-timer from the Nursery says, everything that goes in her mouth is sucked, which makes feeding her a lengthy and unsatisfactory process. The school unit is working on it continually.

The dining-room adjoins the kitchen. There is a part-time cook. When she is off-duty, the nursing staff prepare or serve meals that have often been left ready.

All the children sleep downstairs, in five dormitories. Apart from the Nursery, which is bright and modern, they tend to be gloomy old rooms, brightened by murals on the walls. There are no separate cupboard places for each child: the matron says they would mess everything up and not appreciate it, and she may be right. Clothes are communal, simply graded according to size. The first jumper that comes to hand goes on the first child waiting for one.

The Nursery children are fed in their cots by the girls – invariably a difficult job. There are no drinks at this time. Later, around 3 p.m., I watch the same girls giving out afternoon drinks of tea to the same children. They show great patience, though not necessarily commonsense. John, aged sixteen and severely spastic, flails around, excited by the unaccustomed attention, while his girl attempts to get at least as much liquid inside him as outside. Yes, it would be easier to use a cup with a spout, she agrees, but the nurse gave her this plain plastic beaker. No, they are not trying to train him to an ordinary cup. There is no particular reason. She does not change it for a different cup.

A piece of wood that must be some sort of toy or part of a toy hangs on a string tied to the side of John's cot. It is the only toy around, though he seems to be able to grip. He takes no notice of it, but when anyone passes his cot or looks over the top, he breaks into big grins and becomes very excited.

'We took him out once,' Mrs R said, 'in the summer when we had some voluntary help, and he was giggling and making little delighted noises all the time. We had to find a sort of spinal carriage and he could not see as much as we would have liked. But my word, he did enjoy himself.'

There have been no outings since. John has company now only when someone goes into the room to feed or change him. When that is happening you can hear little shrieks of delight from the Nursery. He is sixteen and a place is being sought for him in an adult Home. Matron is very scathing about hospitals.

Number 5 used to have an upper age limit of eleven, then it was raised by a couple of years, and now a number of children stay till sixteen. One, there from babyhood, is eighteen. Margaret is near the the upper limit, too. A painfully thin spastic child, she sleeps on the only divan bed in the Nursery. She has been in the Home since she was a toddler and becomes distraught if taken out of that room.

She is not without the ability to develop relationships after her fashion. She has become so attached to the six-year-old girl in the next cot that she is inconsolable when the child is taken over to the school for a couple of hours. A teddy bear has to be put in the cot and covered up well enough to deceive the eye, to keep Margaret quiet.

Next door, Nicki is spending the day completely alone in her dormitory while the other children are out. She is fourteen, looks half that age and suffers from fits. She has caused some surprise by learning to walk a few steps.

Nicki is responsive in a babylike fashion. She will hold your hand, laugh, put her long, thin legs through the bars to poke you with her foot as she lies in her cot. There were no toys in or around the cot. I didn't see anyone go to talk to her and the only time she was taken out, despite finding her feet, was when the staff nurse walked her into the Nursery to sit on a chair and have her afternoon drink with the others.

Out from behind the bars, she could sit perfectly on a chair and hold her drink with help.

1.30 p.m.

Over in the Development Unit, there is a free play period. Most of the children are getting about on the floor, on feet or knees or bottoms. One is in a wheelchair, reaching down to hang wooden bricks together – a deafening noise. A girl sleeps through it on a mat on the ground. She is, the teacher says, going downhill physically.

Mrs R taught normal children before coming here two years ago. She thinks it helped her get these children in perspective. She has a different aim for each child. 'Sometimes it is as simple as getting that child to look at me for a moment.'

She has had a fair measure of success and, though aware of their limitations, she would like the chance to 'stimulate' the children in the Nursery. 'Some of these I've got are as handicapped. I don't know what was the deciding factor in which children came and which didn't. I can't see that their fits can be that much more of a problem than any other child's. Most of them can be controlled to a large extent.'

One common factor is that the children in the unit are younger than those in the Nursery, where the oldest boy is eighteen, though he has the body of a baby. He is too old for school, anyway.

There have not always been good relations between school and Home. The school unit is trying to drag the set-up into the 1980s and there is a feeling in the Home that they managed perfectly well before. Mrs R has taken it on herself not only to involve psychologists and other outside experts but to fix appointments for physically handicapped children to see an orthopaedic specialist and to look into their rights.

'They were in old pushchairs that were falling apart and there was no money to buy new ones. Then I found out that with a doctor's prescription we could get a buggy free for each child who needed one. The local GP who comes in to see the children when they are ill just signs a note for us.'

It is hard to see how such basic bits of information are not common knowledge in a Children's Home. There is a Management Committee, made up of local people often with the training to be of use (like the bank manager who audits the accounts), a House Committee, for minor internal problems, and an Appeals Committee. But basically, as in all old-style establishments, Matron rules supreme.

3.30 p.m.

Over in the Nursery, the children are all in their nightclothes – and have been since 2.15. They have been 'up' (i.e., in day clothes) since 7.0 a.m. Short day. There is, as always, a trained nurse on duty to cope with possible medical problems. The old hospital idea that the mentally handicapped need nursing is strong, but perhaps there is also a high availability of trained nurses in the area. The Development Unit assistants have to hold NNEB qualifications, something not stipulated by Education Departments in other areas.

The girls have given the Nursery drinks – not talking to the children or communicating in any way, but rather treating the process as a tricky mechanical manoeuvre. It's that, all right – with the children flat on their backs – but nobody seems to have taught them to make it more besides.

The teacher, bringing back the children, stops for a chat at each cot. The matron, back from a business outing, gives two children a cuddle. Surely you can teach attitudes if they are not contagious.

The girls are waiting for the taxis to call so that they can escort the other children from school. They usually return to a new extension, a large, bare play room totally devoid of seating or furniture.

Their problems, Matron thinks, centre upon the mixture of children under one roof – from the hyperactive to the totally helpless. 'It is much easier to stick to one grade or degree of handicap. All we get offered by the Local Authorities are cot cases, and though I hate to think of them having to go into hospital – and where else is there? – we cannot keep taking them.

'In future we are going to have to take children who have at least a glimmer of potential. We have the Development Unit now. It is only sense to use it.'

The most urgent need, she says, is for 'a big injection of cash'. 'We are always having to scratch and scrape.'

Conclusions

I am not in any position to discuss the quality of life of three-quarters of the children at the Home, but there are obvious ways it could be improved to benefit everyone.

Family units, for instance. A Home this size tends to become a mini-hospital, with none of the advantages. Dividing the children into groups of six or so, with a couple of staff members from each shift taking permanent responsibility for them would give both children and staff more sense of belonging.

I cannot accept that all the girls would find it impossible to look after the Nursery children for any length of time – providing they can do something constructive with them. Or what about dividing the very handicapped among the family units, one or two to each, thereby spreading the load, and providing a stimulating environment for the cot cases?

As far as the Nursery children go, they simply puncture another myth – that smaller, voluntary Homes are more humane towards, understanding and caring of the profoundly handicapped than the other alternative, hospital.

They are less liable to criticism, more resistant to change than the majority of today's hospitals. They can go on propagating bad practices and old ideas without fear of contradiction. Who sees to contradict?

It was not so much the fact of things being wrong that was alarming – but that nobody in charge thought them so. The children were fed and kept warm and clean. True, they have physical problems that would tax the most inventive innovators, but would John be any more at risk if he was taken out a few times a week for a walk around the village in whatever vehicle could be found to accommodate him? And one could be found after a word in the right direction.

Would the children's arms and legs drop off if they were got out on play mats every day and given simple basic exercises taught by the physiotherapist? Physiotherapists in schools and other places are delighted to pass on snippets of skill to untrained helpers. Ten minutes per child once a week – often all the time they can afford –

is useless, if not backed up by reinforcement when they are not there. And look what the child gains in mental stimulation. What a break in the monotony and loneliness.

Bang goes the widely held belief that carers in voluntary Homes – and this one operates under the name of a respected charity – are selfless, dedicated people. I don't think they need be saints and I am not anti-youth, but Homes like this need more mature people among the lower ranks, too. Not just any older person, but those with the experience of life that gives them a natural warmth towards the children. The sort of warmth the younger girls can pick up – or perhaps just learn not to bottle up self-consciously.

This was tried, briefly, but the two recruits, local housewives in their thirties, did not last long. They objected, one staff member said, to 'being treated like kids with no initiative'.

'Someone of this age, with experience of children, will not be bossed around and told how to do every little task. The whole attitude to staff relations would have to be changed. We did have one girl who was really good with the kids. She made bath-time and meal-times a social and learning experience, playing with them, trying to teach them self-care tasks. There were constant complaints from above that she was useless, that she was too slow with bathing and feeding.'

An injection of cash? Yes, it is needed. But an injection of new thinking is even more urgent.

BROOKVILLE CENTRE – A CHILDREN'S HOME

The Brookville Centre is a two-storey, oddly shaped building (due to having begun small and grown piecemeal), standing in a built-up residential area, between a major city and an industrial town. It seems to have no front or back and is quite hard physically to get into, until you realize that there are two doors, ever-open, and you simply wander in as you please, without waiting for someone to answer doorbells or ask your business.

I was given an invitation to come and talk to whomever I wanted at any time – on the premise that the Centre has nothing to hide and much to be proud of. Parents, too, are allowed – no, encouraged – to visit at any time and bring the rest of the family.

It is all very open and might put a strain on the staff who have to get on with the job whatever, were it not for the fact that only a quarter of the twenty-four children have regular visits.

The Centre was opened in its present form, as a residential hostel, in 1974. It was built and is run by a local Fellowship for the Handicapped, which was formed to help the disabled generally, but finally settled on mentally handicapped children as the area of greatest need.

Each child – they are aged between three and seventeen at the moment, but there is an upper age-limit of twenty-one – is sponsored by his local council. This still leaves some subsidizing to be done by fund-raising and involving local firms and organizations. The Centre is very keen on this local involvement of factories, offices and public houses – an excellent idea in a heavy industrial area where friends groups and individuals with time for charitable concerns might be in short supply.

In fact the director puts the successful growth of Brookville down to 'a progressive committee and close co-operation between voluntary organizations, the community and Local Authority.'

The annual budget in 1977 was £80,000 with an average of 22 children over the year and forty staff. When I was there, there were actually twenty-five children – one over quota – and a waiting list. They try to cater whenever possible for short stays.

Brookville is run by a committee of interested people, not parents. The director, who for all practical purposes runs the Centre – *is* the Centre – would not like parents so closely involved because of what he calls their tendency to be emotionally motivated – not just towards their children, but the handicapped generally. The director Mr L, now in his sixties, has been involved from the start.

He is an ex-army man and local councillor, who launched an appeal to raise £20,000 to build the hostel during his year in office as chairman of the Local Authority. His experience with the handicapped previously had been on a voluntary and bureaucratic level when he worked for a local Welfare Department.

He is responsible for day-to-day running, as administrator, and makes decisions concerning the children's training and treatment. He has no training, but is confident that he can rely on commonsense.

'We have a library of books here and people keep coming up with new treatments and sticking fancy names on them. It comes down to observing the child very carefully and working it through its problems. Each child here is an individual and is treated accordingly.'

He is a man of strong views, who prides himself on being a plain speaker. Not everyone finds him instantly reassuring or lovable, but he is an efficient organizer and an energetic fund-raiser.

Parents are often on the receiving end of his bluntness, when he disapproves of their handling of their child. He doesn't, he says, mince words, and whilst some parents appreciate it, others find it too much. One father, whose daughter spent a couple of weeks at the Centre and was well treated, would not send her again, 'because I object to any organization that is run by one man'.

His attitude to parents, which permeates the whole place, passing down to the lower ranks, too, is unsettling. He feels they are over-emotional, over-protective, spoil their mentally handicapped children and let them run their lives without realizing it. A wild generalization.

'The child must fit in with *your* life, not you with *his*. Parents are too soft.' Mr L does not say *all* parents, of course, but the suggestion is strong and it must get through to families, surely, and make them feel under attack. Something that could discourage visiting, the last thing the staff want.

Most of the children come to them spoilt, their only aim in life being to get attention by fair means or foul, he insists. 'Attention-seeking' is a phrase he uses a lot. He encourages parental contact, but when children go home for weekends, Mr L says, they often come back with the same bad old habits the Centre had almost rid them of. 'People make too many excuses. You get parents and grandparents who unconsciously finish every sentence with "but of course she's handicapped".'

Some parents he approves of: one 'because she appreciates what we are doing for her child'.

Mr L dreads the Centre becoming a 'dumping-ground' and hopes that the children with parental contact will, under their guidance, improve sufficiently to go back home to live. When I doubted that families who had made the painful decision to send a child away would reorganize their lives again to accept him back, he was adamant. 'That's where you are completely wrong! The parents will not have to reorganize their lives. The child must fit in with them. Our aim is to make the children capable of doing that and manageable for the families.' If only it were as simple as that.

Mr L knows each child and his background thoroughly, 'although social workers don't always give us full information and we have to find out by ourselves. If only everyone was as open as we are here, it would save a lot of problems.' Social workers come in for even more criticism than parents.

Each child with the comprehension of wrong-doing is punished for bad behaviour. 'If I threaten something, it must be carried out. We had a time when staff used to say to a child: "You won't go out at the weekend for doing that". Then the weekend came and it was forgotten. I made sure the punishment was kept, though it doesn't often happen.

'By knowing a child, you know what punishes them most. Bobbie, for instance, is a very affectionate girl. She can't bear you to be unfriendly. So if she is sent to me for bad behaviour, I simply let her sit in a chair while I carry on working and ignore her completely. That punishes her more than anything I could say.

'One strict rule is instant dismissal for hitting a child. People who work in other establishments are always amazed and sceptical, but I keep my word. A slap the first time might be something a damn' sight worse the next time. So I sack them.'

There are two boards on the wall of Mr L's small office, with the names and ages of all the children and small triangles showing when they have had visits from parents and when their social workers have been in touch. Each child's life at a glance. After each name is the name of a local firm who have 'fostered' him or her. Donations from firms go towards treats and outings for their particular child. It helps to personalize it.

Raising funds is a continual headache, but the Centre has enough at the moment for the committee to buy a large house in Wales for a holiday home, which is let when their children are not using it.

The Centre is divided into two sections, simply referred to as Upstairs and Downstairs. Downstairs, home to sixteen children, is made up of one large, basic playroom, with vinyl tiles on the floor, large, hardwearing toys around and a box of cuddly toys. There is a television, a large, low table where children can play with blocks and Lego; some battered armchairs. It is partly divided from a dining area, with stackable chairs and tables, served by a hatch from the kitchen. The children spend a lot of their time in the playroom. Empty, it looks large. Filled with a crowd of very active children, it shrinks to inadequacy.

At the other end of the playroom are the wash-basins and toilets, with each child's flannel and toothbrush labelled. Opening off the playroom, through a glass door which is kept locked, are the dormitories. These are light and airy, with three or four beds or cots to a large room. Each child has his own chest-of-drawers with his own clothes.

Everywhere there are plaques, declaring that this room was furnished or this item was provided by one local organization or another. It is the same upstairs. Mr L believes that openly declaring your gratitude pays.

Upstairs is quite different. It is a newer part of the building – a vast sitting-room/playroom with modern storage wall units, parquet floors and a three-piece suite. Double bedrooms with their own sinks line two sides. On the other side are the bathroom and toilets. The eight children (six girls and two boys) help with household tasks, and one important function of a newly added small flat is to give them an idea of how to cook, clean and care for themselves.

That is the bulk of the Centre as far as the children are concerned. There is a small play area and a hydro-therapy pool, which even the most handicapped children use. There is a large hall, used for an old people's luncheon club – and available to any local organization, as is the pool. The care staff are not expected to involve themselves in helping with the old people: that is done by another group.

Upstairs and Downstairs could be two different Homes. They look different, they feel different and the children are very different indeed. The sixteen downstairs residents are severely handicapped (though only one is physically disabled), dependent, and often with behaviour problems. Sixteen of them, all together, is just too many, particularly in such limited space, and the atmosphere is frantic.

The eight children upstairs are the cream of the Centre – mostly older, though that is not a criterion. They are toilet-trained, capable of simple self-help tasks and, apart from occasional outbreaks, socially acceptable. Some of them came directly into the section; others were moved from the ground floor when they improved.

A couple of boys from downstairs are being trained currently with this in mind, going Upstairs for afternoon tea on Sunday to improve their table manners. I cannot imagine any of the others reaching this stage, but I am assured they will in time.

Care staff are interchangeable, working Upstairs or Downstairs according to a rota. 'There are twenty-four children and each member of staff is equally responsible for all of them,' said Mr B 'Children can choose favourites, staff must not.'

Next in command to Mr L is Vivien, the nursing supervisor, an SRN who is responsible for the practical running at shop-floor level. She is an efficient, down-to-earth, married woman in her late twenties, who arrived via nursing head-injury cases and spastic children. She was hoping to leave soon to start a family.

She is responsible for all the details, from seeing that there is soap at wash-basins to getting vacuum-cleaners serviced for the domestics; from making sure there are sufficient staff on duty to buying the children's clothes from a chain store that is happy to exchange if they don't fit.

Under her are housemothers, in various grades, down to raw trainees. They are divided into three teams, led by a team leader. The team leader I met was a nursery nurse. The theory is that housemothers learn on the job. Those I met had no qualifications or previous experience. Ideally, there should be two houseparents who are qualified as teachers, but this is not always easy to arrange. When I was there, there was only one, and she was new and had not had time to get to know each child and involve herself in after-school supplementary education.

The three teams work in shifts – mornings, afternoons and nights. At weekends one day-shift does Saturday and the other Sunday. They all live out, so there are no split shifts.

There is a laundry assistant who comes in three days a week and is responsible for washing 1,623 personal items weekly as well as 240 bedding items. There is a secretary and an accounts clerk and two nice, motherly cooks. They work alternate shifts, but both have to come in during school holidays when a cooked midday lunch is required for the children. During school term, tea is sandwiches or a light cooked meal. The supervisor and cook plan the meals and shop at a local cash-and-carry warehouse.

Wednesday 11 a.m. – Downstairs

All is quiet. The children are at school, except for Carl (aged around seven, silent and withdrawn), who is not well.

The housemothers and assistants are tidying cupboards and painting the bathroom. One girl – who started that week and left a couple of weeks later – is taking Carl around by the hand. He wears a riding hat, an improvised replacement for the heavy helmet he used to wear to prevent injury when he falls in a fit. Nevertheless there is a giant bump on his forehead.

These girls are the morning shift. They work from 8 a.m. to 2 p.m. and all day Saturday. The afternoon shift (2 to 8 p.m.) will do all day Sunday. A third shift work nights. Day-shift workers take it in turns, two at a time, to come in at 7 a.m. to help with the breakfasts.

They suffer from the drawback inherent in this sort of shift system. They are rushed off their feet for the hour and a half before the children are collected for school, and from 3.30 p.m. – when they come home – till bed-time. In-between, time drags. They fill in with general duties, turning their hand to anything – from painting the bathroom walls to mending toys.

The supervisor, Vivien, agrees that a split-shift system would be far better – getting staff in for the busy morning hours, sending them home and getting them back again for the late afternoon and evening – but nobody wants to work such disruptive hours. The travelling can be prohibitive. One young housemother, who has been there for two years, has to catch two buses with much difficulty to and from work every day.

In the dining area, two tables are out and six girls sit around mending soft toys and chatting. They are nice, friendly, uncomplicated girls, all between sixteen and twenty. There are a variety of reasons for their youthfulness. Getting them young and training them right is one. The most cynical and probably most accurate reason came from one staff member. 'No one older could afford to work for the wages. They are even less than you get in a Council Home and that is saying something.'

I met only two mature housemothers, forty-plus with older children of their own. There are no men around the place, barring Mr L, who does not look after the children on any basic, caring level. Consequently, the children have no contact with men at all, unless they do at home.

One housemother is leaving soon, to begin nursing training. She is a very organized girl, presently involved in writing the daily reports on each child in a large ledger. Each child's behaviour that morning is commented on in writing by the day staff for reference by the later shifts. This happens every day and Mr L believes it to be an essential part of building up a picture of each child. It covers everything from whether the child has been to the toilet and when, to whether he or she is in a friendly mood.

'I think you can overdo it,' said a young social worker, whose case-load includes one of the children at Brookville. 'I get sent these incredibly detailed reports and I can't honestly see I need to know every time she goes to the lavatory. But if I said that, Mr L would accuse me of lack of interest.'

Sandy, a friendly eighteen-year-old, has been working at the Centre since leaving school. She has been promoted by a series of small wage jumps from trainee to housemother. She knew what she was taking on, having helped at a centre for mentally handicapped children during her last year at school.

Two of the girls are in their first week, still in the probationary period. Mr L starts all newcomers on very low wages – part of the test, he says, to see if they are really interested in the job. During my contact with the Home, spread over a month, four girls started work, but only one stayed. It is, one staff member said, the sort of new staff turnover you have to learn to live with.

One girl was plunged straight into the Downstairs section in the morning, and left the same afternoon. It is not hard to understand with a teenager straight from school. Mr L insists they sometimes get the same reaction from girls who have worked in subnormality hospitals.

'They are used to seeing children drugged into a zombie-like state, so that they will not be any trouble. We don't go in for drugs here and it can come as a bit of a shock if you have been used to children just lying around doped.' It makes you wonder if he has been to any hospitals lately.

Nevertheless, there is no shortage of applicants. He showed me a foolscap page packed with names of the people he had just interviewed to find the current newcomers. One of the staff agreed there are always plenty of applicants – 'but very few are of the right kind'.

The two newcomers on this shift are both nineteen. One dropped out of a teachers' training course. I ask if she thinks she will like this job. 'I hope so,' she says, non-committally. When I next go back, she has left. The other girl, slight and earnest, started a nursing career and had to give up because of illness. Since then, she has worked as a nanny, but this is her first experience of mentally handicapped children. She was, she says, more apprehensive about being with the abler, older children upstairs, than the more handicapped ones, but it was easier than she expected.

Later on, at tea-time, I see her taking the initiative and helping a child with feeding himself. She is spooning pudding at an alarming rate into a child who can feed himself anyway. Nevertheless, she joins in and does not stand aloof. It looks promising. She was still there when I stopped going.

'You either like it or hate it,' Sandy said. 'And you find out quick enough. You are plunged in at the deep end and left to get on with it. You have to use your commonsense. You are not taught much, but you learn.'

It took her a year to become a housemother. Another girl complained that she has been there longer and is still only a deputy. The two new girls have been told that they could be promoted within a couple of months and could be fully fledged housemothers in six. 'It depends who leaves,' Sandy pointed out reasonably. 'We can't all suddenly become housemothers and have no deputies or assistants.'

Mr L says: 'A housemother has to be someone you could safely leave in charge of the children. Some of them will never reach that level. What I look for is brains – not the kind that gets you GCE passes, but the commonsense kind. Someone devoted to the job, but willing to bend and try new methods as they appear.'

Sandy echoes Mr L's philosophy about parents being overprotective and doing more harm than good when they get children home for a stay. The director's views are accepted completely. Some of the parents Sandy knows quite well through their visits, and likes them. 'But a lot of the children are better off here than in the homes they come from.' There is a schoolroom atmosphere, quiet chatter and muffled giggles. Mr L is spoken of rather like a headmaster.

One girl approaches the door of the kitchen next-door and asks the cook for something. 'I can't come in and get it,' she explains, with a roll of eyes heavenwards. 'Mr L has a new rule – instant dismissal if we are found in the kitchen.'

Carl throughout has been wandering about, lying against one person's knees and then another's. 'He wants a cuddle,' Sandy explains, giving him one briefly. He sucks his thumb, but does not play with toys. His usual behaviour is to curl up in a corner, sucking his thumb, completely self-involved.

Nobody suggests doing anything educational with him, though it would be the ideal opportunity with time to spare and the other children out of the way. They carry on finding bits of sewing to do. Carl has soiled his nappy, but nobody seems to notice.

Downstairs – 5 p.m. Tea-time

The dining-room section looks surprisingly small and cramped with sixteen children seated at tables in threes and fours. All of them wear plastic bibs and all but one feed themselves, with a lot of mess and a little help. This is a skill most of them had to be taught and still are being taught as a matter of course each day. It is an on-going lesson.

The food is served, sandwiches first, through a hatch, and placed on a rubber mat in front of each child. There is a team leader (a nurse in charge of each shift team), the supervisor and three other helpers, but nevertheless, the pace is hectic, the whole atmosphere frantic. A dishcloth is permanently on hand to mop up the spills.

June, head down, eats everything at a rapid pace. She overturns her bowl of custard at one stage and it is quickly mopped up, but not replaced. A little mongol boy, soon to be 'promoted' upstairs, eats off the others' plates and trots up hopefully for seconds and thirds. Trisha sits aloof, legs crossed, a disdainful look on her face as she refuses to touch her food.

She is, at seventeen, the oldest resident, and her parents – who take her home for frequent weekends – are delighted with her progress from a hyperactive, unmanageable child to 'a real little lady'. A couple of children have to be helped, a housemother standing behind them, raising the spoon with them.

Ricky, arguably the most difficult child there, given to attacking other children and continuous screaming, keeps leaping up from his chair. Vivien, the supervisor, with an eye on everything at once, sits him down, wordlessly, each time. They are working with him on a behaviour modification programme planned by his school and this means ignoring undesirable behaviour and rewarding good. It is, she points out, almost impossible to implement fully without more staff, unless you are prepared to ignore complete chaos. Finally Ricky slips on spilt custard and it is very tempting to say it serves him right, along with a few other harsh words. But he is merely wiped with a cloth – by now most faces are covered in first or second courses – and replaced in his chair yet again.

It is hard to see how there is time to teach any of them self-help feeding skills at this unrelaxed pace, but many have learnt – parents have verified this.

The team-leader, Sheila, is feeding the most handicapped child, Ross, a dark-skinned little boy of three, who has been at the Centre since he was four months old. He is profoundly handicapped, and it is amazing that he stays safe with so many hyperactive children around.

The staff do tend to carry him about a lot and he is put in his cot very early, before most of the other children have had their bath and are ready for bed.

Feeding Ross is a long, slow business. He still attempts to suck everything and choking is an ever-present danger. The food is dry and there is no drink for him. It seems obvious that a drink of some kind would help, but it is not part of the routine and nobody seems to think of it. None of the children are allowed a drink with their tea because of the likelihood of spillages. It is not until they have eaten their sandwiches, pie and custard and a fairy cake that a glass of orange is offered.

The pace is fast and furious. The helpers need eyes in the backs of their heads and a spare set of hands would help. Afterwards there is a procession of children in twos and threes to the toilet (about two-thirds are partly toilet-trained) and washroom.

Then into the playroom, which shrinks from a large space to an overcrowded one as the children run hither and thither through it. The toys are necessarily unbreakable – large plastic bricks, a rag doll, rubber things. Not one child appears to play constructively and there are not really enough adults to persuade them to. There is a television high on the wall, where no child can reach it. It is on, but there is too much noise to hear it.

Two children fight continually. Another screams and demands that someone turn the pages of a catalogue for him to look at.

'He tends to get most attention because he demands most,' said one housemother, 'but if I stay with him all the time, I'm depriving the others.' There is a teacher-housemother present, a new staff member, still feeling her way.

Mr L told me that the teacher normally takes children away individually to a 'quiet room', for concentrated spells of teaching. This little room boasts a two-way mirror, so that a child can be observed, much expensive recording equipment and specially made educational toys.

The teacher-housemother spent that evening in the playroom trying against the odds to play with one or two children at a time, but giving up finally and turning her attention to tidying up and stopping the fighters beating each other up.

It was one of the areas where there is some discrepancy between what happens in theory and what happens in practice. Each child has a carefully detailed development programme worked out between Centre staff and the School. But with staff shortages and changes, and winter ailments abounding, I never saw any child working on his or her programme.

With handicapped children, though, 'education' has a wide context. Certainly feeding and washing training happened, as a matter of course and every day.

The shift system is ridiculous. There is a staff surplus in the middle of weekdays and severe staff shortages at other times. The official ratio of one helper to three children is a paper figure. Taking account of absenteeism, illness and holidays, it is always less. Vivien always allows for one person away in her calculations. It piles the stress on the others.

One weekend lunch-time while I was there she was telling another helper: 'I will have a proper lunch break today. I've promised myself'. Someone failed to turn up for work. She didn't take the break.

Another discrepancy: I did see two children lightly smacked on two separate occasions, one because she was causing another child distress. Both instances were understandable and unlikely to escalate into full-blown violence – but what about the rule?

Upstairs – After Tea

Upstairs was a haven of peace by comparison. Two housemothers supervise and they are plenty. Tea is over and the children are doing small jobs on careful instruction – putting things away in cupboards and in the fridge, fetching a bucket from downstairs.

Mandy is washing up in a bowl of greasy water, more enthusiastically than effectively. She talks about going on a bus trip. She laughs a lot. Occasionally she talks so quietly that she cannot be heard and a housemother tells her sharply to speak up.

It is worth a slight digression here to talk in some detail about Mandy, as she is one of the Centre's success stories. She is a plump, pretty eleven-year-old, giggly and easy to like. It has not always been so. When she came to the Centre, three years ago, her case-notes record that she 'wandered off, climbed out of windows, cried all night, got out of bed at 3 a.m. every morning, soiled the floor, flooded the nursery and was aggressive'.

The youngest of six children, with a widowed mother who cared but couldn't cope with her, Mandy had been in care for much of her life. Because of her tendency to run away, she had always been confined, even tied up at one place.

A year later, the copious records tell us, Mandy had lost the urge to escape and was 'making beds; changing Jane's pants when it needs doing, without being told; staying in bed till 5 a.m.; helping less able children – and singing'.

Not only that, but her mother is a regular visitor and she goes home sometimes for weekends. Though the family come in for some criticism because of over-protecting Mandy and still getting nervous about the possibility of her running off, they are generally approved of. Her mother, I was told, is very grateful and accepts their better judgement on Mandy. Mr L believes that the child will eventually go home to live permanently, but other members of the staff are less certain that it would work.

What is not in question is that Mandy has improved in every way. But why? Mr L talks of observing her in detail and working out why she behaved in the way she did, then 'working her through her problems'.

'We gave her her freedom, in small doses at first. We showed her we trusted her. Deprive anyone of their freedom and they will run away.'

One very down-to-earth staff member felt differently. 'It was nothing special we did here. Mandy had had a rotten time before. We treated her nicely. I think she would have improved anywhere as long as she was not treated badly.'

Mandy shows me round the big, bright, well-furnished room she shares with Sarah. There is a wash-basin in one corner, with each girl's toothbrush and wash things laid out. Mandy can wash, clean her teeth, get dressed and go to the toilet, with only minimum supervision. Like the other seven children, she helps set the table for breakfast, which is at 7.30 during the week and 8 o'clock at weekends. Two day-staff take turns to come in and help the night-staff get it ready and served.

Some time between 8.30 and 9.30, the school transport arrives. The children are divided between three Special Schools in the area and Centre staff keep in contact with class teachers about what each child is learning. Not that they have much time to continue with it.

Fourteen-year-old Bobbie takes over from Mandy to give me a more extensive tour – of everyone's rooms, including her own, decorated liberally with Starsky and Hutch. She spends some time looking for her tights. She wants to wear them the next day, when she goes home. It is a short trip, just a couple of hours, accompanied by a social worker, but it is regular and Bobbie looks forward to it. Normally over-affectionate, she has sudden spells of aggression.

'When she is good, she is very good, but when she is bad, everyone runs for cover,' said one housemother.

Only one child upstairs is a real problem – and Mr L would disagree with that description. Ann is a dark-skinned girl of twelve. She sits aloof from the others and does not join in their games. She has none of the childlike qualities of most mentally handicapped children her age.

She looks intelligent, knowing. Most of the staff have small scars where she has suddenly, and often inexplicably, bitten or scratched them, but she never reacts to other children with such ferocity. Mr L insists she has improved greatly, is far less aggressive than when she came to them. Her social workers are pressing to move her to a hospital, but Mr L is fighting to keep her, insisting they can cope. 'Can you imagine what her life will be like in a hospital,' he says, 'drugged out of her mind?'

No problems crop up during the early evening upstairs. It is very relaxed. Four children sit around a table, colouring-in pictures. Elaine, an eighteen-year-old housemother with a mentally handicapped sister of her own, sits with them, chatting and helping.

Elaine has been working there since leaving school. She remembers Mandy when she first came. 'She was terrible, always climbing out of windows and running away if you left her for a minute. She's a different child now.'

Mandy responds by loudly demonstrating pig grunts. She has been learning animal noises since an outing to a farm and finds them very amusing. She asks about going on a bus trip and going to tea with her friend from school.

The Upstairs children go to church every Sunday, the local Church of England one, though this is not necessarily their religion. No parent has ever objected and the children enjoy the outing.

They go for bus-rides into the nearest town and on regular weekend and school holiday day-trips in the good weather. Groups of them go riding, and there is plenty of opportunity to swim in their own pool.

An argument erupts at the table between the newest arrival, a Down's Syndrome girl who came in as a resident that week and the more aggressive of the two boys. His aggression tends to be verbal. The girl has taken one of his toys and, under a tirade of abuse, quickly hands it back even before Elaine can intervene.

The new girl has not yet cottoned on to the local code of behaviour. She has been living at home, where – according to Mr L – she has been 'running her parents' lives for years'. She teases the staff continually. I watched her hold out a cup for tea and when the housemother began to pour, pull it away quickly with a wicked chuckle. Told to sugar her tea, she began to pile sugar into the cup, spoon after spoon. She sat opposite a member of staff who was cutting shapes out of card and deftly pulled the card from in front of her each time she began to cut. She was tolerated for a while, then told sharply that the joke was over. It will take her a while to learn to live with other people.

The other boy, Terry, is another enthusiast in his friendliness. He hugs visitors and staff members at every opportunity. Mr L has warned staff not to allow him to do this, 'because it is not socially acceptable behaviour for a fourteen-year-old boy'.

The Upstairs children make their own beds, keep their room tidy, bath themselves with supervision and clean their own shoes at night. There is a small flurry of excitement when Anna, who has been sitting alone in an armchair, tries to bite the second housemother, who is trying to get her to clean her shoes.

The woman struggles to ignore this bit of startling behaviour, but holds Anna at arm's length for safety. The staff talk a lot about 'bad' behaviour being an attempt to get attention and best ignored and this is also part of the principle of behaviour modification. But the rules do not seem to apply to a child like Anna. After a particularly angry attack, she will cry and shake with terror – as if at her own behaviour. A teacher who has known her for years regards her not as retarded but mentally ill. Nobody seems sure where she might fit in. She has been in care since she was a small child. Tonight's reaction was sparked off by being told to clean her shoes. Eventually she does as she is told, still alone.

Mandy, undeterred by it all, as are the other children, is off to dress up with her friend Sarah. They return in long dresses and large hats – Mandy liberally painted with eye shadow and lipstick.

She realizes that a kiss can leave a neat red mark on Elaine's cheek and proceeds with great giggles to try to do this.

The team leader comes round with medicines in egg-cup-sized containers, mainly for the children prone to fits. They all gulp it down without complaint, including Anna. Mandy licks the last drop out of the bottom.

She wants to see me out and walks with me to the top of the staircase. 'We wouldn't have been able to let her do that a year ago,' Elaine says. 'She'd be off.'

Downstairs – 6.45 p.m.

'Crossroads' is on the telly, but nobody watches. The playroom looks less crowded now. It is bath time and children in twos are being taken through the dormitory to the one bathroom.

Two women – one a part-timer who comes in for these two hours – are busy in the small bathroom. Starting with the smallest child, Ross, who is now safely in his cot, they work their way up to the two biggest girls.

The door to the playroom is, as usual, locked. A few of the children wait near it for their turn. It seems to be a time of high excitement. The small boy and bigger girl, who were fighting and pulling each other's hair earlier, are still at it. 'His mother keeps asking about the scratches on his face,' exclaims one housemother, 'but however you try to separate them, he keeps going back for more.'

June, who has lived in Children's Homes all her life, climbs up any adult she sees standing – 'almost as if you were a tree and she was a little monkey,' someone said.

She has improved since coming to the Home. She can feed herself and is toilet-trained, but has what can euphemistically be called behaviour problems. They are all, the staff say, desperate attempts to get attention at all costs. She spends a lot of time lying prone behind doors that open towards her, with her fingers in the right position to get caught beneath them.

She will deliberately mess her bed. 'I feel I ought to like June more than I do, said one of the housemothers, 'but it's hard to, when she does such awful things.' She would probably benefit greatly from individual attention – some of the staff think she is the most responsive child they have in the downstairs section – but where could a family or individual be found to look after her?

They are bathed two at a time, three pairs before the water is changed. Some have their hair washed and it is rinsed with a bowlful of water from the bath. Their clothes are thrown into a linen basket – they are changed daily – and they are dressed in pyjamas and dressing-gown, and disposable nappies, where necessary.

Those who have not had their hair washed are taken straight to bed, apart from a few night birds who stay awake late and disturb the others if put in straightaway. Mary, one of the older housemothers, is in the playroom with a hairdryer, blow drying the wet heads. A hairdresser comes in regularly for trimming sessions.

Only one other staff member is around now, the teacher-housemother who is clearing away scattered toys before the night staff take over at 8 p.m. Helen went home at 5 p.m. as usual, having made hasty arrangements for a local lady, who can come in in emergencies, to do so. The night team were short-staffed, due to illness.

At 7.30, there is only Trisha left unbathed, and she is getting quietly frantic about her turn taking so long, pacing the floor. In all probability, Trisha will go on when she reaches the upper age limit to an adult hostel being built by the Council nearby. So will the other older children eventually. It is considered a good area in making provision for the handicapped.

The room is quiet and tidy. Only a couple of children are up. Most of them wake early in the morning, around 5 or 6 a.m., so they are ready for bed early. The staff breathe a sigh of relief. It has, as usual, been a fairly exhausting few hours.

It is the Centre's proud boast that they have only ever turned down one child, as long as a place was available. I have heard this explained cynically by the fact that social workers (referrals have to come through the Social Services) know what child will be unacceptable and would not refer them. But a look around downstairs confirms that this is one voluntary residential unit that does not take the easy-option children.

It is possible the opposite occurs. That children who are basically too difficult for a small home without trained staff, are taken on as a challenge. Anna, for instance, of the unpredictable attacks. Does she really fit in, or is her social worker justified in finding a more secure environment, where more sophisticated treatment is available?

'They can be very tiring down here *en masse*,' Mary says. And then she unconsciously echoes the argument against anything but home or small family units. 'You know, it is only when there are a lot of them they seem so bad. There is not one child here you could not cope with on his own.'

Upstairs – Lunch-time during the school holiday period, shortly after Christmas

There have been some changes. A wall between the main room and a small flat, previously used for a caretaker, has been knocked down. This flat can now be used for dining and cooking and washing up.

Apart from the convenience of no longer having to carry bowls of water up from downstairs, there is an opportunity to teach the children the skills of home-making. There are also plans for bedrooms in there for the two boys, since one of them has started to show an interest in sex.

That is the good news. The bad news is the atmosphere, which is gloomy and tense. The children have all been away for some part of the Christmas period – the one child who could not go home spent Christmas Day with one of the staff – and are unsettled. Both boys are loud, aggressive and swearing.

Sarah, always the most clinging child, cuddles an old teddy bear calling him over and over the name of her little brother. She cries continually, clutches at each adult present, calling for 'Mummy'. It is this very demanding behaviour that drove her parents to find residential care for her. It has improved, but staff complain that after visits home, she is back to square one. One of the boys is driven to giving her a hefty smack. It does not improve matters. The staff are trying to keep them busy with little tasks, until the routine is established again.

Downstairs

Not all the children are back yet. There were only ten left over Christmas, mainly those who have no contact with their parents. One housemother is in charge while the supervisor and team leader clear up after lunch, mopping the floor in the dining area. They are short-staffed again, some people are ill and nobody seems certain who will show up at 2 p.m.

Ricky is being particularly trying, screaming continually, demanding that the house-mother sit beside him, turning the pages of a catalogue (mail-order catalogues seem to be basic playthings). He wants to go out – he is used to going out for a walk or into the playground for a while in the afternoon during school holidays – but there are not enough staff on duty to take him.

Sweets are given out. One little boy gets a toffee stuck in his teeth and begins to shriek. Another throws toys over into the dining area. Hilary mops around them and tries to ignore him. Behaviour modification can be very trying.

As usual in such situations, the quiet ones are left to get on with it. The demanding children, whatever principle you are trying to stick to, are very hard to ignore.

Conclusions

I went to Brookville well aware of the strong feelings of most parents and some professionals that only small units can function happily – but not entirely convinced. Brookville convinced me.

Upstairs, with fewer, relatively able residents in plenty of space, works a treat. Downstairs is, if I may use the word, bedlam. These sixteen, overactive, sometimes disturbed and downright difficult children need more, not less, space and smaller, not larger, groups. Sixteen into one (playroom) won't go.

Downstairs at Brookville has no advantages I could see over the hospital's children's ward, with its ten beds. In fact the atmosphere was more frantic and less homely, and the majority of the children were more agitated and distraught. This cannot be accounted for by claiming that all children in hospitals are heavily drugged. It is not true.

Brookville, however did have the edge in its liaison with the children's schools, which staff took seriously. Programmes initiated at school are, when time permits, continued at the Centre. Even if this only extends to self-help skills like toileting and feeding, which can be fitted into the essential daily routine, it is very important and recognized as such.

It would be hard to fault Upstairs – except where it suffers from faults common to both sections, like staff shortages and high staff turnover. Downstairs would benefit initially from more space, so that the group could be sub-divided into three or four mini-units for day care, each with its own play/living-room and its own staff.

I may be over-sensitive here, but I would like to see a change of attitude to parents. There was a strong anti-parent feeling, all the way from the top down through the ranks, which ranged from condescension to outright disapproval. Not aimed at anyone in particular, you understand, just all of us as a homogeneous clump.

It is a case for junior staff meeting more parents and more professionals from outside who come into contact with parents, and then being allowed to form their own opinions. More open-minded training from outside agencies would help.

THE ELM ROAD FAMILY

It is labelled simply Number 16 – a large, detached house in a leafy suburb. Upstairs live four working nuns who follow their own occupations during the day. Downstairs is home to the Elm Road family, as they have named themselves.

Jim and Eileen Rowe are both twenty-seven. They have three children of their own – aged eight, seven and eighteen months – and four foster-children, all mentally handicapped. These four boys range in age from five to seven; in degree of handicap from moderate (Peter) to severe and withdrawn (Sam). In-between are Roddy who had severe behaviour problems and Khmrain – a five-year-old Asian boy who was believed to be blind when he came to them a year ago, but proves not to be. Khmrain is the child Eileen most regrets not having had there earlier. She is certain she could have helped him greatly and believes she is doing pretty well now.

The Elm Road family may not be unique, but they are certainly rare. It is an experiment in residential care, a cross between fostering and a small children's home, a family unit in the true sense.

The unit was set up three years ago under the auspices of an Order of nuns. The Order financed the conversion of the house, provided all the necessary furnishings and fittings to cope with a decidedly extended family, and found the young house-parents through a national newspaper advertisement.

The Rowes were not, on the face of it, the ideal applicants. An older, experienced couple had been envisaged, with perhaps teenage children. One of the Sisters involved with the project says they chose, finally, by instinct, and perhaps divine providence or plain common-sense guided them, because the Rowes with their energy and enthusiasm do seem to be decidedly suitable.

They are not Roman Catholic, but describe themselves as 'low-key Christians'. Clearly specific religious convictions would not have had much relevance, anyway, with these children. They had no prior experience in this field – both had worked in offices. What they did have was a burning desire to 'opt out of the rat-race and do something useful'. Unlike a lot of similarly motivated individuals, they got the chance.

Eileen did take some short courses during the first three months after landing the job, but mostly they have learnt by experience. As they point out, they are not alone: they have always had back-up from the modern Special School the boys attend and from social workers. They do not, they insist, suffer the isolation natural parents are often heir to.

It helped that the first child to come to them was Peter, a curly-haired six-year-old of Afro-Irish parentage, who fitted in beautifully. He has never been a problem and their baby daughter was a few months old before the other three boys began arriving. The baby was an unexpected addition and one they feared might lose them the job. Now, in many ways, she adds a lot to the family feeling.

The boys came from Children's Homes. All were already in care, without parental contact, and this has made it easier to absorb them into the family. Strictly speaking, Eileen is employed as a house-mother and Jim is free to follow his own employment, but in practice it involves far greater commitment than that from him. Both of them think of themselves as full-time parents to the children, committed to looking after them into adulthood. Jim says: 'To us, this is a twenty-year-project. We will not take on a second batch. It would be like a second family.'

The four boys are brought up as brothers to their own children. They live, eat, sleep and play together. They all go on holiday in a converted motor caravan and have been as far afield as Majorca and Yugoslavia, braving the inevitable stares. The Rowes say they are immune now to the attentions of the purely curious. At the same time, they feel they can do a good public relations job for the mentally handicapped generally and particularly for the Elm Road idea, in which they believe implicitly. They would like to see it copied elsewhere.

Jim has to play a positive role. It would be impossible for Eileen alone to get the whole family up in the morning and have them dressed, fed and ready for the school taxi. The same goes for bedtime, and his presence is essential to family outings at weekends. Because of this, Jim has given up his accounting job and now works part-time and is planning to go to university to study Social Administration.

A lot of his free time is spent taking round a film he has made of the family to schools and groups, giving talks. This is in the interest of raising some of the ten per cent running costs that have to be found after the Social Services have made a grant for each child.

He believes above all in bringing up mentally handicapped children alongside normal ones in a family setting. 'Our children automatically teach the others to do things. The handicapped boys learn from them in a way they never would surrounded only by children like themselves. Peter in particular tries to copy everything. He gets a bit frustrated sometimes when he cannot keep up, but his behaviour is getting more normal all the time.'

Number 16 is a spacious house with enough room generally for seven children – though perhaps the handicapped boys could spread comfortably to two bedrooms instead of all sleeping in one large room.

There is a big lounge/dining-room with television, as comfortable as any home. The furniture is new and stylish. The living-room floor is carpeted, except for the dining section which has vinyl covering to match the kitchen that opens off it.

The kitchen has all mod cons and they're very necessary, too. Eileen operates as a housewife with a large family in addition to her specialized teaching tasks. She does the cooking, washing, mending and ironing, but a domestic help comes in for two hours each week-day morning to do the cleaning.

There is also a part-time care assistant, who comes in from three till six on school days to help Eileen with the children's programmes, worked out at school, and stays to lend a hand at tea-time. By that time, Jim is home to help with bath-time and bed-time. The same woman, incidentally, takes over the children one day each week while Eileen and Jim have their time off.

The boys' bedroom-cum-playroom is at the end of the hall. There is a big cupboard just outside the door, with all their clothing in it, labelled with their names and their colour tag. Each boy is 'colour coded' in this way. All his belongings, including face flannel, dressing-gown and towel is either in 'his' colour or has the appropriate coloured tag for easy identification – by child and helpers.

The bathroom, with toilet and shower, is next-door to the bed-room. The bath is a special deep model and there are wooden steps for climbing into it, plus temperature-controlled taps, so that no child, however adventurous, can manage to scald himself.

The Rowes sleep in a room off the hallway, close enough to hear the boys in the night, though all now sleep well. Their eight-year-old daughter shares a room with the baby and the seven-year-old son has one to himself.

'We have to remember to leave some time for our own children,' Jim said. 'It is a good idea for them to have a room of their own where they can be alone to read or play when they want to. We worried a bit that they might be affected by the situation so we kept in close contact with their teachers. The only reports of them being different we have had is that they are keener than most to help other children at school.'

There is a big garden with swings and a swimming-pool. Fine for summer, but in winter the Rowes are thrown back on their own resources. Eileen averages fifty-four hours a week working and playing with the handicapped children. During school holidays, when they are at home all day, this reaches sixty-nine hours.

Two or three times a week she goes into the school to work with the children and liaise with their teachers. This has occasionally caused a little friction. Working with Peter on a language programme, she was accused of 'going her own way'.

'He had advanced beyond what they were asking me to teach him,' she explained. 'I know what he is capable of, so I worked out what to do and went on to the next step. Obviously I know him better than anyone else.' It is the sort of situation familiar to any natural parent.

Thursday 4.30 p.m.

Eileen is in the bright and tidy kitchen, cooking beefburgers, peas, corn and mashed potatoes for the children's tea. Emma, the baby, is quietly removing pots and pans from a cupboard on to the floor. The Rowes' two older children are down the hall in their rooms. In the living-room, the four handicapped boys are sitting aimlessly. Khmrain is peering out of the french window, his nose and hands pressed against the glass, into the deepening gloom. It is one of his favourite activities. Roddy, who usually clutches at guests and tries to climb on to their laps, is disinterested. He has not been well at school and is, Eileen says, not himself today. Only Peter peers round the open door of the kitchen with a cheeky grin to check on the company.

It has been a hectic afternoon. Eileen's assistant could not come due to illness, but fortunately Jim finished work early and was home to help with a shortened version of the children's programmes when they were brought home from school at 3 p.m.

'What worries me most,' Eileen said, 'is what would happen if we both suddenly went down with something. There have been times when I've felt pretty bad, but I've forced myself to carry on. The Sisters can't help much – they are often out till seven. They baby-sit for us in the evening if we want a night out, but what we need is another resident assistant, who could be on call for emergencies.'

'We hope to bring in two more mentally handicapped children,' Jim said, 'Girls, this time, under five years old because that is when you can help them most, and preferably only moderately handicapped to balance the others. But perhaps we should wait and see about some extra help first.'

Tea is nearly ready. Jim takes the boys to the bathroom, brings them back washed and toileted, dresses them in plastic pinnies (made by Eileen) and sits them at the long, pine refectory table, with his own two children. The baby, in matching bib, sits beside the table in her high chair and Eileen serves the meal and returns to the kitchen to deal with the sweet, while Jim supervises.

It is a surprisingly civilized meal. The boys use cutlery correctly and without apparently great effort, skills they learned since arriving. There is chocolate blancmange to follow, then cups of tea with a slice of home-made cake and iced shortcake biscuits, also made by Eileen.

It is a silent meal, because none of the handicapped children, even Peter, talks. He listens, though, when the Rowe children chat among themselves. The other three are self-involved, except for Roddy, who glances intermittently at the adults.

'He's strange about food,' Eileen said. 'Sometimes I cannot get him to eat his own meal, but when the others have finished he snatches up any scraps they have left. I can't understand him.'

5.30 p.m.

Tea over, the boys are sent down to the playroom, while Eileen and Jim clear up. I follow them down. Emma, released from her chair, toddles after us.

'We worried a bit about bringing her up with the boys because people said she might copy them,' Eileen had admitted. Emma has not done so, though she obviously enjoys the company of her foster-brothers and accepts them. Why not? They have always been part of her life.

Eileen and Jim explained to the other two that they would be getting 'four new brothers who could not do all the things they could.' Jim said: 'We did not go into the technicalities at that stage. They just accepted. Children do.'

In the playroom, Khmrain sits on the floor, turning the pages of a book with little shrieks, happy in his own world. There are plenty of toys around, but the boys do not, on their own, play with them.

Sam lounges on a bed. He is big and slow-moving and still somewhat withdrawn. 'He's just like Muhammad Ali,' Jim had said earlier, wrestling with him and getting a rare smile. 'When he first came here, he wouldn't move a finger to help himself. Now he can feed himself and dress himself – slowly, but he does it eventually.'

Peter, ever sociable, brings a book for me to read to him. Emma squeezes in beside him and they both listen. They play together a lot. In some ways, they seem close to the same mental level, but Eileen says that Peter acts the big brother sometimes, looking after her and teasing her.

A page has been torn from the book. Peter points to Emma, shaking his head in disapproval. There is little he seems not to understand. When Eileen, busy in the bathroom, shouts for him to fetch the nappy bucket, he takes off at the speed of light. He thoroughly enjoys helping. What singles him out most is his sociability, but it also puts him in a funny in-between position. Integration is not always automatic.

You can see him struggle to keep pace with the older Rowe children. He is very vulnerable, totally dependent on their good nature. Mostly they let him join in, but sometimes, like any children, they get a bit fed up and want to play more sophisticated games without him. Later in the evening after Peter had had his bath, I saw an incident that perhaps illustrated the point.

In the living-room, while the others were being bathed, the older children sat at a table, playing at 'dining out', drinking imaginary champagne out of little vases and pots. Peter arrived as soon as he was bathed and became very agitated, trying to join in and snatch a vase for himself.

'No, no,' said the girl, 'you'll only break it.' But Peter's non-verbal demands continued and he got a vase – which sure enough, he put down heavily and cracked.

'You naughty boy,' said the girl in exasperation – and Peter managed to look puzzled, ashamed and disappointed all at once.

6.30 p.m.

Eileen starts the baths. Emma is first in. She is left in while Peter and Sam join her. They undress themselves – Peter quickly, Sam very slowly and with a great deal of verbal encouragement. Eileen and Jim are both in the bathroom. Sam needs a wearing amount of encouragement and gentle bullying to get him to wash himself.

It would be so much simpler to undress and wash them, but it would defeat the object. Making them self-sufficient is the whole point of the exercise. It has been a non-stop daily training routine since the boys arrived, working to a programme that is carried on at school – and it has worked. They have acquired skills it is hard to imagine them learning in that space of time in a hospital or a Children's Home.

Toilet-training is a case in point. None of them arrived completely trained. Working to a behaviour modification programme, Eileen was told to take them to the toilet every half-hour, rewarding success, ignoring failure. It didn't work. There were too many failures. Eileen stepped up the bathroom trips to every five minutes. One of the severely handicapped boys became completely toilet-trained in two weeks. The others soon followed suit.

Emma sits nonchalantly in the middle while two of the boys join her in the bath. Roddy is moving slowly and reluctantly. His stomach upset has kept him close to the toilet for most of the evening. Every so often he gives small, unhappy little cries.

Bathed, his hair washed and in his dressing-gown, he follows me into the playroom/bedroom. He is a good-looking little boy, with a sad, desperate little smile, which he directs always at adults and mostly at women. That he has behaviour problems is not surprising. He was an only child, severely epileptic (this is now controlled) and apparently close to his mother. Then his parents' marriage broke up and without warning his mother left him at a play-group held in a general hospital and refused to take him back. She has disappeared and has not contacted him since. He spent a year at that hospital and was then moved to a short-stay unit where his behaviour veered between refusing any contact and clinging desperately to any familiar figure. He was considered severely disturbed, though eventually the familiarity of the surroundings reassured him.

Another year passed and he was uprooted once again and moved to Elm Road. However desirable the new home, it was still bound to be another traumatic experience. He was, at the time of arrival, a demanding, possessive, aggressively jealous child with a constant need for physical affection. He would scratch and bite any child that an adult showed an interest in.

Hardly the ideal child to join a family with a small baby. Someone who worked closely with Roddy at this time doubted – and indeed still doubts – the wisdom of the move. He should have gone, she insists, to a family where he was the youngest if not the only child; where he could be 'the baby' and be helped to grow out of his insecurity.

The ideal and the possible are often two different things. Roddy's behaviour, however, has definitely improved. Perhaps being plunged into this household was a baptism of fire, forcing him to learn more control. Or perhaps he has gradually realized that these people are here to stay.

There were bad spells. At one stage he would attack Emma and they had to be kept in separate rooms. He is over that, but when he saw the baby on my lap, he tried to push her off and curled up with his head against my shoulder. At other times he would push between Peter and me, pinching Peter, trying to drive him away. Peter, of course, just fought back.

There is something very touching about Roddy's search for affection – but it must be wearing to live with. The Rowes insist they did not realize how bad his problems were until he was part of the family, although they had visited his school and the short-stay unit. They have the option of turning down a child who does not fit in, but have not yet used it. Where teaching self-help skills is concerned, they have succeeded well with Roddy. One thing rankles – he never looks happy.

7 p.m.

Roddy is still giving intermittent little shrieks and Jim, with the first show of irritation I have seen in either of them, shouts at him to shut up. The child glares resentfully.

A few minutes later, he tells Roddy to go to the toilet. Roddy clings wordlessly to the door, refusing for a long time to budge. Finally he gives in sulkily to a very determined command.

Jim Rowe says that they do, when necessary, give the boys a smack – 'exactly as we do our own'. They are also, as punishment, sent to their room alone – a very effective method of punishment, the Rowes say.

Tempers are getting a bit short all round. Peter pushes shut the door of the bedroom just as his older foster-sister is coming in and catches her bare toe.

'Say you are sorry,' Jim tells him. Peter approaches the girl, stares at her for a few moments, then bursts into tears.

'All right, all right, I think you've apologized,' Jim says.

There is just enough time for a final play session before bed. All the children plus Eileen and Jim troop into the living-room to skip round playing 'I wrote a letter to my love', followed by a brief spell of barn dancing to the family's Country and Western music. They try to do this every night, but Jim admits that 'sometimes we are just too exhausted'.

The normal children and Peter thoroughly enjoy the session. The baby sits smiling in the centre of the dancing circle, miraculously missing being trampled to death. The three remaining boys tend to lift their feet off the floor when you hold their hands and try to sit down. They seem rather confused by it all.

7.20 p.m.

To bed, with nappies for three of the boys to avoid accidents. Nobody has thought to tell Eileen where she can buy plastic pants big enough to fit Sam – the sort of simple information professionals forget – and she has been squeezing him into the biggest baby size and wondering what to do next.

Jim does the rounds, having a final little chat with each boy, giving them all a goodnight kiss. Roddy turns his head away and buries it in the pillow.

The older children are ready for bed. The baby has only to be put in her cot, then Jim and Eileen are free to go upstairs for a House Committee meeting.

The House Committee meets once every two weeks, to discuss everyday problems. Generally three of the Sisters are present, plus the head teacher of the boys' school.

The handicapped boys are left in their beds while the Rowes go upstairs. They have given up getting out of their beds after months of being firmly led back to them if they wandered. On the agenda for tonight's meeting are the new curtains Eileen wants to buy and the possibility of changing the kitchen floor covering, as well as a general chat about the progress of each child.

Normally Eileen buys such items as clothes for the children and gives the receipt to the Committee for repayment. She is economical with money and time. To save both, she cuts the children's hair – very professionally.

'You have to learn a lot of new skills in a job like this,' she says. 'You become a medical expert, too. I'm very good now at knowing exactly when to call a doctor and when to treat minor complaints myself.'

There is also a Management Committee, which meets quarterly and includes a teacher, a psychologist, a consultant psychiatrist, a schools inspector – though not all the members turn up. This group covers long-term issues on policy and spending and the Rowes are expected to make a full, official report.

7.30 p.m.

All seven children are in bed, before they make their way upstairs. Eileen has not eaten since I have been in the house. She is small and fragile and looks very tired. (The first time she answered the door to me I was ready to ask if her mother was in, when she introduced herself.)

She finds the job tiring, she admits, and aims to be in bed by 10 p.m. on most nights. – 'It is harder than office work, but much more rewarding.'

The children's clothes are laid out neatly for the morning. Mornings are even more hectic and have to be planned to the minute. At 7 a.m. Eileen and Jim are both up to get the handicapped boys out of bed. They wash and dress themselves with supervision and lashings of encouragement. 'It takes eight minutes per child for them to dress,' Jim says, 'on a good day.'

This done, Jim starts breakfast. Eileen calls the two older children if they are not up, sees to the baby, has a shower and gets dressed herself.

She takes over supervising breakfast, while Jim gets ready for work, if he is going out immediately. He drives the older children to school and the handicapped children are ready and waiting when the school taxi arrives at around 9.15 a.m.

Six Months Later

A care assistant had just been taken on – to live upstairs in the flat recently vacated by the nuns. 'There will now always be two of us in the house with the children at a time,' Eileen explained. Jim was due to start his university course in the new term. A room upstairs had been converted to a study for him – and a place to get away from it all for the two of them on their days off – distant enough not to be too worried by commotions downstairs.

Have the changes made a difference to the basic situation? Eileen thought carefully. 'I think, obviously, it will take us one step further away from the idea of just being a complete family. It is no longer just mother, father and the children – but it was necessary.'

Jim does not agree. 'The new helper lives upstairs, completely separate from us except when she is on duty. It is very little different from having someone come in at busy times during the day. Lots of normal families have mother's helps.'

They had reached a stage, they agreed, where something had to give. 'We could not see ourselves going on for more than a couple of years without help.' Jim admitted. 'We had under-estimated the demands on our energy. You've got to remember this is experimental. We have nothing to go on. We are learning all the time.'

And the two additional children? 'We have decided on one more as the maximum we can possibly take,' Jim Rowe said.

Conclusions

Against fairly heavy odds, the Elm Road family works. Perhaps, given the right mix of children, foster-parents and support agencies, it should – but that mix is elusive. Everyone is crying out for family units for children in care, and this, surely, is the ultimate in family units.

If there is an obvious fault, it is the lack of community involvement in a situation where it should exist. True, Jim gives talks to local schools and pupils raise money, but they do not – and I am sure they would if invited – come in and play with the children or take them out.

Contact with local people is remote. The children are rarely taken out locally. Too many children and not enough hands, Eileen points out. It is a quiet, refined area. No camaraderie in the corner shop or gossip over the garden fence. So, the children are hardly known in the neighbourhood. Perhaps, in view of the fuss that blows up in similar places when a hostel or home is planned, a low profile was thought safer. Mainly, I think, it is simply that the Rowes have neither the time nor the incentive to go soliciting neighbourly interest. There are many, more urgent things to see to.

Elm Road is a reversal of the norm. The children have been taken into the family home, instead of the houseparents going out to work in the Children's Home. It is a hybrid system with no official name yet. It could be called simply fostering on a large scale, were it not for the fact that the building was provided and adapted and a committee oversees the project.

None of the children has regular parental contact. If they had, that might put a different complexion on matters. Certainly it would introduce new conflicts of trying to please families as well as everyone else involved. Eileen admits to being shaken when she found the mother of one of the boys on her doorstep with a social worker. She would not mind parents visiting, by arrangement, though she doubts she would actually welcome it. 'We like to think the children are *our* family. It works better for them and us that way.'

The first essential ingredients in the success of the Elm Road family are the Rowes themselves. I have heard criticism of letting a completely inexperienced couple with family commitments take on a group of mentally handicapped children.

They might not have the time to give, they might be unreliable as a long-term bet, the critics said. Or, almost as bad, that as non-professionals they were likely to be sentimental, unrealistic do-gooders. 'The sort of people who say "ah, poor little thing" about every mentally handicapped child and then go off them when they find out they kick and bite and soil the bed,' was how one experienced professional described not the Rowes themselves, but her idea of a couple who might be attracted to such a job.

The Rowes however, seem quite the opposite. Intelligent, down-to-earth with just a touch of forgivable optimism. Eileen, for instance, hopes that by the age of eighteen, all four children will be self-sufficient enough to live in a Group Home caring for themselves. Apart from Peter, it looks a forlorn hope.

Have they bitten off more than they can chew? There are signs of this – Jim's realization that he is needed at home more than a full-time job allowed him to be; the need for additional staff; the couple's acceptance that two more children would make the load too heavy. I see it more as coming to terms with reality. Dedication does not solve every problem. They will continue to need every scrap of support available from statutory services, if they are not to find themselves under the same strain as normal parents – multiplied by four.

Eileen, perhaps because she is closer to the everyday problems, was very aware of the need for time off and somewhere to spend it – other than the same floor of the house, where they could hear every noise and never really relax. Being on duty round the clock is a very exhausting business, as any parent will verify.

The Elm Road project is, in many ways, an experimental unit. The Rowes have had no guidelines to go on and have had to learn by experience. If they cannot, in the long run, do things quite the way they set out to, it is not a sign of failure. Hopefully, their experience will have made the going a lot easier for anyone brave enough to follow.

Whether adding extra staff and perhaps more children, will dilute the strength of the project remains to be seen. It would be a pity to go on expanding until it ended up just another Children's Home.

At the moment, what the Rowes have in abundance is enthusiasm. You can only hope it will not be allowed to die or be buried beneath the mountain of problems they are bound to encounter as the years go by. While they keep it, it is worth years of cynical experience.

5

Voluntary Agencies – Provision for Adults

THE MANOR – GIRLS ONLY

Five miles out of the nearest town; half-way down what was once a quiet village street and is now more of a through road for speeding traffic, you turn left into the Manor. The driveway winds through a wooded portion of forty acres of land surrounding the building. You follow a sign saying 'Craft Shop', and suddenly you arrive at the house itself.

Tall and grey and grand, with a heavy door, it is almost gothic in appearance. You pull the bell rope and there is a distant jangling echo and the deep baritone barking of a large dog. You half-expect the door to be opened by a tall, dark man with barely concealed fangs, followed by the Hound of the Baskervilles.

Instead, after a long wait, Bill F, who is dark but far from menacing, arrives. 'I thought I heard the bell,' he says. 'Why didn't you push it open. It's not locked.'

The Manor is a home for the mentally handicapped in the old tradition: an isolated community. Thirty 'girls' between the ages of sixteen and fifty live within the protective, enclosed atmosphere of the 120-year-old building. 'The Convent', a wit at another home called it. It has been a voluntary home since 1952, when the family who owned it – parents of a mentally handicapped child themselves – decided to put it to good use.

Ironically, their child was a boy, who died before he got the advantage of it and the Manor became a Home for Girls. It had close ties with the Steiner Homes, but the ties have loosened. The only reminder is morning prayers – and perhaps the very fact that it is a single-sex establishment.

Today, it is the clear product of the couple who took over its running seven years ago, and put their stamp on every facet. They do not call themselves 'manager' and 'manageress' or 'houseparents', but simply Maggie and Bill. A young social worker remembers

Maggie's horror when she, on her first meeting, called her 'matron'. 'We have no title,' Bill says. If anything we would like to be called 'Mother' and 'Father' – we like to think of the girls as a very large family'.

Bill is a quietly spoken Scot, an ex-engineer and one-time professional footballer. Hence his description of his role and philosophy as something like Brian Clough's! 'He takes players with bad habits and smashes them down, then builds them up from scratch. We have had to do something like that here.'

He doesn't think of his change of job, from engineering in the Middle East, as all that surprising. 'It was a supervisory job, so is this.'

Nevertheless he came to the job with the advantages and the disadvantages of no experience and an open mind. So did Maggie, his wife. Her only qualification was of bringing up three children from her first marriage; the eldest was born with spina bifida.

'The advert asked for a mature woman – and I was certainly that,' she said. 'There is no way of knowing if you can do a job like this without trying it. It is not a matter of qualifications. You either can or you can't.'

They arrived at a place, which from their description, had not moved far out of the Dark Ages. 'The girls would sit around crying in corners, like babies. They had been treated like babies, so they behaved like them,' Maggie said. 'When they met us in the hallways, they would cower. They did no work, except an occasional bit of art, painting the same childish pictures day after day. If they felt like it, they could do some weaving, but they were given the choice and girls like these you have to encourage and bully a bit.'

I have not only their word for the Manor of yester-year. Helen, now in her forties, is what Maggie and Bill describe as a junior staff member (the only full-time one apart from them). When they came she was a resident, a fact hard to account for. There would be no question of her being sent to a Home for the mentally handicapped nowadays.

Helen gave a hair-raising account of the old workhouse atmosphere, with no male visitors, even brothers; no books, television or radio, plenty of floor-scrubbing for the more able, and unkind treatments all round. 'There was nothing to do in your spare time. We spent most of it in bed.'

Brenda, one of the more mentally able residents, who can read and write, has spent twenty-five years in the Home. 'We've had some people looking after us who were not kind at all,' she said. 'Maggie and Bill are the nicest people who have ever looked after us.'

Someone running a home like the Manor can be – possibly has to be – something of an autocrat. There is a lot of responsibility, a lot of power. Bill is aware of this. 'People like our girls are pawns. People in authority use them as stepping-stones up the career ladder, or to perpetuate their own ideas.'

There is the awful fear of the sort of damage a strong-willed person with all the wrong ideas, could wreak. These are not allayed by Bill's explanation that though a Local Authority inspector calls every six months, he always gives a week's notice first. 'Ridiculous,' said Bill. 'You could organize a big show in that length of time. They should have *carte blanche* to walk in at any time – and they should take advantage of it.'

There is in fact a ruling body over the Manor, a board of directors associated with the original family who started it, but they do not live on the premises and only deal with the administrative side.

The girls' happiness and comfort then lies with the resident houseparents or whatever you care to call them. The success or failure of such places – and there are still many of them – depends on the right people finding their way to them. An uncertain commodity, these Right People.

Bill's and Maggie's joint philosophy in a nutshell is that busy people are happy people. 'Everyone is better in harness,' Bill says. They set about creating activities for the residents, planning a regular daily work schedule. Some of these projects were ambitious, like candle-making. Experts doubted that they could teach mentally handicapped women, even allowing that many were – to use that annoying but descriptive term – high-grade.

The idea was to turn the Home into a workshop-cum-residential establishment, keeping the residents occupied, whilst giving them a pride in achievement. If, incidentally, it helps support the Manor in a small way, so much the better. That is secondary.

Bill says getting their idea accepted was a slow business.

'We had to persuade the directors that a craft shop was a good idea and that people would come out here to buy from it and that the girls could do it. Previously the girls were only taught whatever the particular houseparents of the day knew about. At one stage there was a great interest in the garden. I got them to employ staff – experts in their own field – to teach.'

The craft shop, the first part of the house you see inside the door, is proof that it can be done. It is open for part of every day and all day at weekends, when it does a great trade with passing motorists out for a country drive.

Cane wastepaper-baskets, trays, patchwork cushions, tapestry, woven oven-gloves, pottery figures and lots of other items are labelled 'I helped to make this', – with the name of the girl. 'You see, we don't lie. The staff may have to help with the finishing off,' Bill said.

Tuesday 10.30 a.m.

The shop takes up the sizeable hall and one small room. Apart from the goods made in the Manor, there are other, bought-in, 'crafty' items, from rocking-chairs to jewellery. It looks good and gives the visitors more choice. The girls tried making jewellery once and though they managed, it was not a popular seller so they gave up. The same goes for candles. They gave up making those, but managing it was an achievement. 'It takes ages to teach some of them,' Bill says. 'Then when you have lost all your patience and are just about to give up, it clicks.'

The shop is the only part of the home the casual shopper sees and it is out of bounds to the girls. Maggie and Bill are happy to show groups of people around the Home, though, by arrangement – and provide teas to supplement funds. The girls love visitors.

It is one answer, they feel, to the criticism that residents in these old-style Homes have no contact with the outside world. 'The world comes in to them. We get a lot of visitors. Groups in coaches, some schoolgirls come regularly and a young wives' group from the village.

'Of course,' Bill adds wryly, 'you could criticize that, too. The zoo syndrome.' The girls, in return, get invitations to amateur shows, and the like. They were out as a group four times over Christmas.

A young woman pops her head around the screen that divides the shop from the Home proper and enquires if Bill is going out.

'Back to work. You shouldn't be here,' he tells her sharply, and she goes. 'She was a real little animal when she came here,' he says, 'and look at her now. The difference is incredible. You have to be firm. You have to be aware of them as people, so that you know when a smack is the right punishment and when it is the last thing you must do because it will make that particular girl withdraw inside herself.'

Behind the screen is a beautiful old house, that has seen better days. It's a bit run-down and seedy. The decorative floor tiles are uneven, but the oak panelling up the sides of the wide staircase looks as good as new.

Battered chairs and settees line the lounge. There is trouble with peeling plaster, rising damp and worn lino here and there. Upkeep must be dauntingly expensive. All finances are dealt with by the directors and the girls' fees (they have recently had to be increased to £1,500 a year) pay the bills.

Most residents' fees come half from their Social Security allowances and half from their Local Authority. (The girls come from all parts of the country. One even comes from Brazil.) Only six are part-private, their parents paying the Local Authority share.

At this time of the morning, they are at work. Bill shows me into a small room, with ten girls seated at three tables, some doing tapestry, some knitting, some busy at meticulous patchwork. Only one teenaged girl is too handicapped both mentally and physically to join in. She is putting shapes in a nursery post-box.

Pauline, the needlework teacher, comes in three days a week. The girls call her by her Christian name. They are very friendly, overwhelmingly so in some cases, perhaps because they see so few outsiders. We have novelty value. The work is impressive. Pauline gets out a tapestry cushion in complicated design which would put an expert to shame.

This is a piece of work by Caroline, a haughty, articulate young lady in her twenties, who looks normal, talks articulately and stands out from the others – the round peg in the square hole.

'She is one of the girls visitors go to first,' Maggie says later. 'Seeking out the most normal face, you see. People tend to do that. Oddly enough she is one of the girls we have had most problems with. She attended a normal school for a long time, then something went wrong.'

In the pottery room another group of girls are fashioning dollops of clay, some with natural skill, some not so well, all enjoying it.

Their teacher shows me their current prize piece – a model of one of Maggie's three black labradors. A quieter group this – they do not shoot so many questions. The groups rotate – everyone having a go at everything. Pottery, needlework, weaving, basketwork. Corny, old-fashioned, traditional stuff, but these girls enjoy it. They are articulate enough to tell you if they don't.

The four specialist teachers come in three or three-and-a-half days a week and, if Bill and Maggie have a week off, will come in overnight on a rota.

'We used to have terrible trouble with staff,' Bill says. One wrong person here can do a hell of a lot of damage. The staff have to do things our way or the girls get confused. They feel instinctively if someone is not right. They are not educated out of instinct. If they don't like you, they say so.

'Maggie and I never managed to get away for a fortnight's holiday until last year. If we left them with residential domestic staff for a day, we would come back to find them ten degrees under and all our work gone to waste. We don't bother with resident staff now, except Helen. You get odd people. Some of them just want to hide away from the world.'

Today, the weaving teacher has not come in, so there is a group at a loose end in the sitting-room. Bill shows me around the large weaving room, with its looms standing shoulder to shoulder. They look complicated enough to puzzle the average Mensa member but, with a couple of exceptions, the girls can operate them.

The designs they are working on vary from simple to highly complicated. Vera, the oldest resident, a spastic in her fifties, turns out delicate baby blankets. She and a few of the other old hands can set up their own machines.

'Oh, they are lovely girls,' Mrs N the weaving teacher, in her seventies, told me another day. 'I have quite a long drive to get here, but I would miss them so much if I couldn't come.'

The teachers range in age from their thirties upwards. All are women. Bill is the only man they see regularly, apart from a seventy-year-old gardener. One very quiet mongol girl in her twenties whispered conspiratorially to me, 'I have a boyfriend'.

'Oh,' said the teacher in charge of that group, 'they took a fancy to one of the men who came on the trip to Spain with us. They all think he is their boyfriend now.' The Manor has taken part for the first time this year in a Local Authority scheme to take the more able individuals from Adult Training Centres and hospitals on holiday to Spain.

Bill regrets the fact that it is a one-sex establishment for one reason.

'I think the girls would be on their best behaviour to show off if we had some boys. We are frankly behind the times here. We are not geared to take men. It would need building alterations and we would have to think about introducing contraception. These liberal ideas worry me a bit. If a mentally handicapped boy forms a relationship with a girl and then it breaks up, does he understand he cannot do that with just any woman he takes a fancy to? I don't think our girls would be wanting to jump into bed with anyone. They are interested in men. If I've been nice to one of them, I'm her boyfriend. It is platonic and childlike, not sexual.'

And then, in the next breath: 'We used to have a lot of masturbation to deal with and what I would call platonic lesbianism. Since they have been busy, that has died out.'

The work rooms, except for the weaving room, open off one long corridor. There is a small all-purpose room between needlework and canework, directly opposite the kitchen. Maggie is in here, doing a spot of hairdressing.

They have tried having the girls wash their hair themselves, but it didn't work. Now Helen shampoos in the kitchen and Maggie trims and blow-dries across the way.

Maggie is firm but motherly. 'You get so involved with these girls,' she says. 'We used to find we were never off-duty, working from first thing in the morning till late at night, seven days a week. We try to go upstairs to our flat at 6 p.m. now and Helen sees them off to bed.'

'But we still find one of us will make a remark about a particular girl – and we are awake half the night discussing her problem. They have changed terrifically from when we came. Each girl does her share of the work. It almost runs itself.'

'We had no set programme to change them. We just were ourselves and made it clear what we liked and didn't like. Some of the younger ones will even give a bit of lip now. It's great, remembering how cowed they were.'

Bill pops in and out. He is supervising lunch today – he and Maggie take turns – with a group of the girls cooking it.

Monday 11 a.m.

Maggie and Bill have taken a weekend off. They are due back in the afternoon. Kate, a young social worker who first came to the Manor as a schoolgirl volunteer and became a friend, is in charge.

'I see a lot of residential places, but there is something about this place,' she says. 'Maybe I'm prejudiced, but it seems to have a nicer atmosphere, it gets into your blood.'

Helen, inevitably, is busy. 'Helen could run this place on her own now,' Maggie said to me on one visit. It is not a meaningless compliment.

Every Monday morning, Helen takes a group of girls upstairs to clean their bedrooms and bathrooms. The six upstairs rooms are enormous, with four or five beds to each without crowding. More like dormitories, really, with five bathrooms between them. The clothes for each room hang in a communal wardrobe, with no front. There were fitted sliding doors but they kept coming off, Helen explains.

There is little privacy, no stylish decor, but the rooms are comfortable and adequate. Each bed has a duvet, paid for – on Maggie's instigation – by the girls, out of their pocket money allowances. They make their own bed; except for two who cannot manage without help.

The girls don't get pocket money in their hand. Maggie and Bill think it encourages pilfering. They have seen it on visits to residential hospitals, they say. Besides, there is no place to spend it. Only two of the girls go out daily – to the village to collect newspapers and small essentials. Helen occasionally takes two or three with her into the nearest town, just for the outing or to buy clothes.

They can ask to have something bought out of their allowance. Brenda bought herself a lamp and a bedside cabinet recently. Or rather, they were bought for her – she didn't go out and choose them.

There is a small quietroom-cum-sickbay, with a single bed, for anyone who might disturb the others in the night or is not feeling well. There is nobody medically qualified on the premises, but then none of the girls need nursing. A doctor can be called in from the village.

Each bed has a pair of pants folded neatly on top of the cover. Helen, in charge of the laundry, washes pants every night, so that they have a clean pair daily. She changes sheets once a week and on Thursday evenings before tea, the girls change into dressing-gowns and everything washable is fed into the automatic machine and tumble dryer.

Helen is paid £6 a week. Yes, it does seem gross exploitation but, she says, in the past she did the work for nothing. She is happy, she insists. Officially she has a day off each week, but she doesn't usually take it. Old institution habits die hard.

'I can come and go as I please any day, so what is the point of having one set day off,' she asks. 'I go out when there isn't much to do. I go to the shops. Sometimes I take a couple of girls with me and we have tea.'

Doesn't she resent all those years of normal living she has lost?

'No, but sometimes I look back at the way things were and think, "did I really put up with that?" '

She wears jeans and a polo-neck sweater, a slim, ordinary-looking woman in her early forties. She has a slight physical handicap, which was worse when she was young and probably accounts in part for why she was sent here.

Could she live and work outside? I am sure she could, but I doubt that she thinks so. What would happen if Bill and Maggie were to leave is the big question? Would she have to revert to her former status? Bill thinks she would choose to live with her sister and that she has built up the confidence to do so.

Helen's bedroom, with all her own possessions and a television set, is down a hallway, apart from the others. Bill and Maggie have their flat in that wing too.

Downstairs in the roomy kitchen, Kate is supervising and trying to remember where they order cakes from when it is someone's birthday, as it is today. 'We're the kitchen wallahs,' says one of the girls amiably.

Caroline, who works fast and efficiently and can cook a meal from scratch, shows some irritation with the other, slower girls. The next time I visit, she has been sent to bed early for making one of the kitchen girls cry.

'She can't leave people alone,' one of the other girls offers by way of explanation.

Dinner is at 12.30, half-an-hour late. Kate has placed me between herself and a quiet, smiling girl called Pauline. There is roast beef, potatoes and cabbage, following by a dish of tacky rice pudding, for which Kate takes the blame.

There is orange squash on the table and the girls help themselves. One girl serves each table. The teachers sit together, at one table. There is a genteel boarding-school atmosphere. Pauline has an orange instead of rice pudding, because she is on a diet. Maggie keeps a check on weights. Pauline doesn't mind – she has pudding at weekends, she says.

She tells me about her two little nieces. The girls don't talk to each other much over lunch. Pauline's conversation seems to be more by way of politely entertaining the guest. 'Their table manners put the rest of us to shame,' Kate says, 'they are very, very proper.'

Rosemary, one of the few with no family contact, lays the tables and clears up. She has a perpetual worried frown, broken only by an occasional smile when she meets your eye.

In the old days, most of the girls arrived automatically from a small voluntary Children's Home on reaching sixteen. Nowadays entry is via an assortment of avenues, but vacancies are rare. Put bluntly, there is usually only a place when one of the residents dies. They can be choosy in finding the right girl to fit in. Everyone comes on a three-month trial. 'I prefer to see someone come in from a subnormality hospital,' Kate said, 'because I know how awful conditions are there and this is going to be such an improvement for her.'

Thursday 6 p.m.

Supper is over. They've had boiled eggs and bread and butter, with biscuits and cake to follow, and sweets for an extra treat. Rosemary is tidying the tables, the washing-up wallahs are crowded into the kitchen, and the three black labradors are romping about.

Bill has 'flu and he and Maggie have retired for the night. Helen is in charge, doing the rounds, keeping an eye on things.

I am greeted like an old friend by half-a-dozen girls and interrogated in the kitchen by Shirley whose method of holding a conversation is to shoot questions in her cut-glass, top people's voice. She never forgets a fact or a figure or a face. 'I sometimes think Shirley is on the borderline between subnormality and genius,' Kate said. 'She has a computer for a brain.'

Shirley is forty and has been there since the Manor opened. 'Guess what?' she intercepts, in a lull between personal questions. 'Daddy has a new car, a Daimler. What do you think of that?'

Brenda is another one of the 'originals'. She attended a normal school for a time, and explained haltingly to me how she could not keep up with the normal children and they used to call her names. 'There are a lot of things I can't do. I can't always understand people.' Would she not like to live outside and perhaps go out to work? The thought horrified her. 'Oh no, we are safe here.' She is nervous and quiet, much given to reading her Bible, and she is sensitive to other people's feelings. 'Do you mind if I ask about your little boy?' she enquired tactfully.

'You are interested in these things, aren't you? You do want to hear?' she asked, half-way through telling me about her youth, searching for the right words – and, slowly, finding them.

Brenda is the sort of handicapped person – capable of reading, writing, communicating and looking after herself in a limited way – currently being encouraged to live semi-independent lives, in hostels and Group Homes.

She would hate it. Perhaps with a different background, she would have adapted. And perhaps not. She is not one of life's flamboyant souls, anyway, and now she is full of fears of the outside world. Men, in particular, worry her – the result of a frightening adolescent experience and the dire warnings of her concerned parents about the dangers of 'strange men'.

Should we feel sorry for her? Has she missed out? Brenda has status in her quiet way. When I asked one of the younger and more voluble girls a question, she would call Brenda. 'Brenda will know the answer,' she'd say, confidently.

By 6.30 we are all gathered in the sitting-room, the numbers divided between two television sets (one black and white, one colour) at opposite ends of the room. The same programme is on both.

Television used not to be allowed in the Manor. Now Bill worries that the girls watch too much of it. 'They get so much more out of television than us, though,' he says. 'They hate violence. If there is anything unpleasant on, they switch off the set.' In fact they go to bed so early that most of the programmes they see are of the 'family' variety, making self-censorship unnecessary.

In the sitting-room, there is a natural pecking order of kinds. The older residents and the more capable and talkative younger element, like the kitchen wallahs, are at the far end in front of the colour set. I sit with them because they are the ones I know. Not that I singled them out – they came forward from the start.

When they are all together you can see the vast differences in ability and personality. There are only about a dozen of these confident, highly social girls. They just sound like more. The others sit quietly, doing nothing (though there is a cupboard full of games and books), watching the proceedings or withdrawing from them. One young girl plays patience at a table, ignoring the company and the television.

The leaders and the followers, as in any walk of life. Nevertheless it worried a friend who came with me – the mother of a quiet handicapped woman, who might have fitted in there.

'There isn't enough supervision,' she said. 'I bet the quiet, less capable ones get bullied by the others.'

I saw no sign of it, but I was surprised to find them spending the evening without supervision. Helen was down the hall in the staff room and looked in a couple of times.

Bill said there used to be some bitchiness when they first came. 'We couldn't leave them alone together. It isn't like that any more. If anything does happen, you can bet some tattle-tale will come and find us and let us know.'

'The girls themselves are very rule-conscious. Newcomers are quickly made aware of what is acceptable and what isn't. I think it is best to let this code of conduct come from the shop floor, so to speak. You take it better from a workmate than from the boss.'

A visitor creates a certain amount of excitement. Photograph albums were brought out and pressed into my lap with half-a-dozen running commentaries going at once. It is rather like being in a classroom full of enthusiastic seven-year-olds – but no children were ever so proud of their families, particularly young nieces and nephews. Only the older hierarchy keep quiet and aloof from the photograph album stampede.

When a baby appeared on the screen, there were a lot of 'aahs'. Frustrated maternalism or a feeling for all things helpless? Usefully it extends to helping the less able around them. The most handicapped teenager is also slightly spastic and has to be helped to feed herself. It is one of the most sought-after jobs, and you wonder if a few more severely handicapped girls would not be more of a boon than a burden to the girls. But that would demand more staff.

Families are encouraged to visit – some come a long way and stay a couple of days in the village – and to have the girls home. Most do, though some of the parents are old now. There are official parents' meetings twice a year.

Bill and Maggie, like almost all those in charge of residential Homes, have mixed feelings about parents. 'I get on with most of them,' says Bill. 'But put it this way: if I had the choice of a girl from a hundred miles away and one from ten and both were equally acceptable, I'd take the one who did not live locally. I don't like parents dropping in all the time. It is disruptive.

'Let's face it, we are bound to have differences of opinion with parents. We are telling them how to treat their children, we all think we know best.'

I ask Diane, a tall, energetic thirty-one-year-old to tell me what she has been doing today. Her Thursday, like most of her weekdays, went like this:

7.00 a.m.	Get up, wash, make beds, say prayers
7.30 a.m.	Jobs – clean toilets, put clean pants out for next day. Go downstairs. Spread butter on bread for breakfast. Do serviettes
8.00 a.m.	Breakfast
8.30 a.m.	Go to village with Linda
9.00 a.m.	Classes (sewing)
10.00 a.m.	Coffee break in dining-room, then back to class
12.00 noon	Dinner, then jobs – washing up, serving staff coffee
1.30 p.m.	Back to classes – dancing in hall in the grounds
2.30 p.m.	Coffee break – then class until 4.00 p.m.
5.00 p.m.	Supper – then evening jobs to be done, before watching television

Dancing has just been re-started after a long break when they had no teacher to take this class. It is something they do on Saturdays, too. Otherwise weekends, especially when it is not warm enough to go outside, tend to be dull days. Some of the girls go to church in the village, but they don't have as good a relationship with the church as they would like, Bill says.

In general the villagers know and, in a limited way, mix with the residents – occasionally inviting a couple of them for Sunday tea. 'We had to seek people out, though,' Maggie said. 'I went round talking to people, knocking on doors, inviting people to come to the Manor for coffee.' Again, it is probably the sociable and socially acceptable First Eleven who get these perks.

Thursday nights are particularly popular for viewing. Everyone likes 'Top of the Pops', though with varying degrees of dedication. When Brenda tries to continue talking to me in a whisper, there is a loud 'ssh' from the younger ones. When a sturdy young lady singer comes on and I remark that she could do with one of Maggie's diets, it almost brings the house down. A good place to be a bad comedian, the Manor.

The situation comedy that follows is much appreciated, then at 8.30 p.m. the girls rise *en masse* and say goodnight. Now I understand Brenda's surprise when I asked her if she doesn't get hungry before bedtime since their last bite to eat or drink is at 5.00 p.m.

Helen is in the staffroom, with the dogs, watching television. She is alone, no longer one of the girls, but with nowhere else to fit in. A limbo existence. She is not lonely, she says. She will see that all the girls are asleep before she locks up and goes to bed herself. She has to be up early in the morning, as every other morning, to get the girls organized. She would not like any more help. She has seen too many failures.

9.05 p.m.

The heavy door clangs shut. Helen goes back to her rounds. Outside is completely black and silent. Inside only a few lights remain on and there is not a sound.

Impressions

The Manor is the sort of old-fashioned, isolated residential community that goes totally against current trends. There are many people who would like to see such a place closed down and the residents absorbed into the community. The Local Authority are currently pressing for the girls to go out daily to work at the nearest Adult Training Centre, quite some distance away.

Bill is against this, though it would make his work-load lighter. 'The girls do far better and more satisfying work here with their own teachers than they would do at a Local Authority centre. I've seen those places and the staff do more of the work than the trainees because there is pressure on them to show results. Our girls would gain nothing from going out.'

Maggie, more involved with the personal care of the girls, does not believe in the fend-for-themselves attitude of putting more able people into Group Homes and boarding-houses. 'They need supervision to maintain the standards you set. There has to be authority, someone to remind them to do things, otherwise they just go downhill.'

Bill is more cynical. This business of getting parents to keep their mentally handicapped kids at home until the parents die or are too old to cope; all the talk of keeping them in the community: it's more to do with money than the wellbeing of the handicapped.

'Those are the cheaper alternatives. I prefer to get girls when they are young and adaptable. What forty-five-year-old mongol can really fit into the community, when she has never known anything but home till her parents died. They have difficulty fitting in anywhere at that age, even here.'

Maggie and Bill are convinced that their way is the only right way. They have to be to cope with such a demanding and financially unrewarding job. They estimate they would earn £3,000 more each year between them working for a Local Authority in a similar capacity.

They couldn't stand the bureaucracy, they say – 'all that filling things in in triplicate and having to report every little event'. The Manor to them is not so much a job, more a way of life. The freedom to do things your way has obvious attractions.

One of their biggest fears is of someone who does think very differently taking over from them eventually and 'changing everything without regard for the girls'.

I asked Bill what qualities are necessary for someone running a home like the Manor.

'Awareness,' he said. 'You have to know the residents and know when they really mean something and when they are trying you out. Everyone thinks they have this awareness but they don't. It takes time to learn. I was here over a year, before I knew a true story from the other kind. I took one girl to the dentist three times, when there was nothing wrong with her teeth, before I realized she was looking for attention.

'In these days of higher education, we are taught to believe what we hear, but with our girls you have to look more deeply and believe what you see. The other quality is leadership. You have to be head of the family. But there are different ways of leading different people – and that's where awareness comes in again. To be honest, I don't like talking about qualities. Ideally a job like this – to do it well – is something that should come naturally to you.'

I think the Manor works because of the people who run it, the fact that they have been there for a relatively long time and the stability that brings.

There is continuity of routine. Days are pre-planned down to the last five minutes, so life is consistent. For these girls, that is vitally important. Yet there is an unhurried, un-neurotic atmosphere about the place. A naturalness in what by our standards is a completely unnatural set-up – a one-sex, segregated community. The girls themselves do not suffer from it. Those who do talk are outgoing and friendly.

Little things niggle. Is there sufficient supervision in the evenings and at weekends? Wouldn't a couple of men on the day staff redress the all-female balance a little? (But then, where do you find male needlework and weaving teachers?) Shouldn't the residents be given a regular sum of pocket-money each week and the opportunity to spend it as well as to save it? It would be a positive reward for work, a bit of independence and they are bright enough to appreciate it. Shouldn't they see more people, have a change of scene, go out to the Adult Training Centre?

The system can only function with so few care staff because of the number of fairly able residents who can do their share of the chores and do not need special attention. There is no hardship in lending a hand in the efficient running of your own home. As Bill points out, we all have to do a bit of housework and for these girls – more than most people – it gives a sense of belonging, of being useful.

'I tell them, "do your job, then you can do what you like".'

It is relevant that perhaps a third of the residents are older women, in their late thirties or forties, and came from a childhood spent in an exclusive and caring, but strict residential home. They are used to authority, discipline, a certain amount of isolation.

The young girls are, on Bill's admission, cheekier, more independent and need to be treated differently. The next generation of high-grade mentally handicapped girls will have led even more independent lives and may well find the days of patchwork and early bedtime no substitute for the mixed company and the noise and excitement of teenage clubs and adult centres. They may have to look harder to find the right girl to fill the Manor . . . or make some fairly radical changes.

CHADWICK HOUSE – A SHELTERED COMMUNITY

It would be a churlish parent indeed who would ask for a better setting for his handicapped son or daughter than Chadwick House.

The large, L-shaped Cotswold farmhouse is set in eighteen acres, with outbuildings for farming and craft activities, and has been modernized sufficiently inside to make it thoroughly comfortable without spoiling its beauty.

There's even a wishing-well, filled in and planted with flowers for safety, to catch the eye as you crunch your way across the gravel-covered courtyard to the pine door with its shiny brass knocker.

Thirty-one people between sixteen and twenty-nine live here, twelve women and nineteen men. They are accommodated in three- and four-bedded rooms, three two-bedded rooms and two single rooms (proudly occupied by two 'older residents' in their late twenties who had spent several years previously in another Home in the group – and whose parents are very involved with fund-raising).

The rooms are furnished pleasantly, most with new furniture, some with elegant old pieces from other Homes. It is a new Home – it had only been open a year when I was there – so there is little wear and tear. Everything is smart and new. The manager and manageress, Mr and Mrs G, are a childless couple, who fall neatly between the rigidly professional and the untrained parent figures.

Mr G – the staff, though not the residents, call them by their Christian names – is a trained nurse who has also worked on the administrative side of a hospital. One previous job involved him visiting mental handicap hospitals to make reports on conditions, and this, he says, is what made him want to run a place like Chadwick, 'where I could use the good things I had seen in other places and discard the bad, the institutional ideas and attitudes'.

Mrs G is no mother-substitute. She is far too young and attractive. Her day, she says, is taken up mainly with managing and running the place. What she does have, though, is an almost unique ability to talk completely naturally to the residents, who are fairly high-grade, but nevertheless mentally handicapped young people.

How many people *do* talk to them without condescending or making painfully obvious efforts at displaying equality? Mrs G has the knack, and she and her husband are sufficiently sophisticated to be acceptable to the parent and the 'Friends' groups who raised £150,000 to buy, convert and equip the house.

Chadwick House and indeed the Trust that runs it and (to date) four other agriculture-based Homes, are undeniably middle-class. Parents tend to be involved, informed professional people who have sought out the possible alternatives for their children and decided that this is the best.

Mind you, not everyone who comes to that decision gets the opportunity to do much about it. Between all the Homes, there is a waiting-list of eight years and the central office gets 700 enquiries a year. As the Homes are, in theory anyway, partly self-supporting, the ability range demanded is high. All but two or three residents in each have to be 'contributors', able to work on the farm, the garden, in the house or the craft shop.

It has been argued that each Home could support double or treble that number of non-contributors, the more severely handicapped – and that the abler residents would enjoy helping them as part of their duties. But that would demand a lot of re-thinking on the part of management, staff and parents of residents already settled in.

Families with reasonably capable sons and daughters might object to them being mixed with the more handicapped. There is a great deal of parental sensitivity in this area. Not only facilities but attitudes in the Homes are geared to a high degree of independence among residents.

It is heartening to see the number of families actively involved at Chadwick House (even though one breakaway village community is reputed to have been started by an ex-employee mainly to get away from the hassles of parental interference).

At Chadwick parental involvement on management issues is taken care of at parent/staff meetings held every three months. I attended one of these, which packed the dining-room, people travelling from all over the country.

'I hope you are not going to write anything controversial,' warned one parent-committee member, which promised interesting things. In fact all that was discussed was fund-raising (with thanks for that done and encouragement to do more) and, with the help of a guest from head office, the future direction of the Homes.

They have recently formed a Housing Association, which gives access to government money for building purposes. There was talk of opening one new Home each year to try to accommodate more from the waiting list, and of building small satellite homes in the grounds of the main ones to take the more independent in small unsupervised numbers.

'I think parents like that idea but they want to know where *their* child fits in,' Mrs G said afterwards. And there did seem to be some vague uncertainty about the fairness of creaming off the best for possible special treatment.

One father informed me that he sat on the Council, an administrative body of the Trust and would see to it that parents' views were represented strongly on these issues.

Parents asked about mixing up ages for a more even balance in future. It is obvious that while you only take residents up to twenty-eight years-old, you are going to start out with a healthy, appealing crowd of youngsters as at Chadwick, and end up with a geriatric unit. This has started to happen at one of the early Homes, where there has been a lot of premature ageing among residents, necessitating a Special Care Unit being tagged on, employing nursing staff.

There are plans in the future to move people within the Homes circuit for a good balance, the guest reassures. Then he says a few words about the need to look anew at assessment procedures and the demand and the possibility of mixing some highly dependent cases with the very capable – of varying the handicaps in each home. 'They are often better at helping each other than we are at helping them.'

It is promising but vague. Parents and staff drift off to tea and sandwiches in the next room and their children join them. Twenty-one-year-old Pippa's parents, who used to do a 600-mile round trip to see her before she was transferred to Chadwick House, are pleased with her new home.

'She wants to come home to us less now and she is eager to get back,' her mother says. 'That is how it should be. This is her home.

She has a boyfriend here – a romantic, childlike relationship. I don't think there is anything sexual in it, but he is important to her.'

Is there anything else they would like to see in the Home? They both want more teaching – better facilities for further education, as opposed to work training.

Twenty-year-old Jill's parents apologize for being boring but cannot think of anything they would want to improve. 'She is happy, doing interesting little jobs.' Jill was away at a special boarding-school. Their Local Authority thought she could be accommodated very well in their Adult Training Centre when she left school and refused to foot the bill for her to come to Chadwick House. The family, who have been involved for years with fund-raising for the Trust, pay a portion of the fees. Jill is one of the few who have to be subsidized.

Most residents are paid for by a Local Authority: eighty-five per cent of the necessary £62 per person per week comes from that source. Parents are asked to make a donation and encouraged to involve themselves in fund-raising. What happens if they turn mean or unwilling is not stated – and fortunately most don't.

Rather like the building society principle, where years as a saving member stands you in good stead when you want a mortgage, families with their eye on a place would be wise to involve themselves in fund-raising from the first enquiry. There are sixty 'Friends' groups, forty-five of them very active. Regular national appeals are mounted and publicity sought. It is all run in a professional manner from two centres. The grand scale of the Homes and their rapid growth makes it hard to remember that it was started in 1962 by a group of concerned parents who wanted to see their children settled for life.

Is this, then, the sort of residential establishment that parents, allowed the luxury of choosing, want for their children? How galling for the modernists – who want the mentally handicapped living in and depending on the community – that what these places resemble are the colonies of the early part of this century.

The colony was set up to offer facilities, care and segregation – though more for the good of the community than the mentally handicapped initially. There were residential units – a school, a hospital, usually a farm on one site – so that the residents could be self-supporting and occupied.

They fell from favour for many reasons, but the upsurge in the last two decades of village communities or agriculture-based Homes like Chadwick shows that there were some points worth salvaging and parents in particular recognize this. They don't all want their sons and daughters thrown in the deep end; to sink or swim as part of normal community life. They simply do not believe the world is a kind enough place to help them make it. They want them sheltered.

Wednesday 11 a.m.

In the entrance hall, beautifully clean and shiny down to the sealed, stone floor, a domestic help is vacuuming rugs. Jan, one of the residents, is dusting the white-painted banisters. For an old house, it has a surprisingly light and airy look. It is warm, freshly painted, newly carpeted, very much the desirable residence from anyone's viewpoint.

Some of the residents are out swimming, taken in the mini-bus. Outside the front door J, who is a gardening instructor, and two of the boys are weeding. Neil is a mongol and fairly talkative. He recently attended a conference where the mentally handicapped themselves gave their views. A nice idea, but Neil, one of two speakers from Chadwick House, cannot unfortunately remember what he said. He enjoyed it, though.

J studied fine arts – an incongruous background – but he is well up on gardens, and staff seem to be picked more for themselves than for their training.

There is a lot to be done with the gardens, good though they look. They had not been touched for years. One problem for J, working through them gradually, is that he is not sure which team of workers will turn up to help on any given day. Sometimes it means abandoning the day's plans and turning to easier jobs, more in keeping with the workers.

Residents choose which work they want to do – garden, farm, the house or crafts. Normally, they stick with that choice for the week – and in practice the bulk of them keep permanently to indoor or outdoor jobs – but there are some change-overs.

The biggest differences are seasonal. The girls are notorious for preferring the great outdoors when the sun shines and turning into home-bodies when the temperature drops. Some of the boys, too.

Would it not be simpler to allocate jobs according to need? 'Not really,' J says. 'They won't work well if they are bored or unhappy. When that happens, you might as well down tools and go in for the day.'

Another difficulty has been finding tasks that do not turn out to be more trouble than they are worth. Could they cope with milking cows, for instance? They are trying goats to find out.

So far there is a nanny and a kid who has to be fed several times a day. It is a job that requires a lot of patience and gentleness and proved too much for the residents. Still, the goats are popular, as much pets as a source of produce at the moment.

Neil's favourite job is collecting eggs from the hen-house every morning. His £1.75 pocket money – the same amount is put away for each of them each week – is spent mostly on pop records. On Saturdays a lot of residents go into the nearest town, either on the bus with a staff member or in the Home's transport.

Across the yard, at the back of the cottage where Mr and Mrs G live, Tom is clearing ground for fruit bushes, a new project. At twenty-nine, he is tall, wiry, well-dressed in a 'young gentleman-farmer' style. He invariably looks scrubbed, shaved, and immaculately turned out, even in wellingtons!

Tom has been in one of the more distant Homes since he was a teenager. His widowed father runs a farm in the next county. He was taught by tutors and never went to school – enough, you would think to make him remote and unsociable. In fact he is quite the opposite, inclined to take over the duties of host, showing visitors around and giving them a rundown not only on his own family, but everyone else's.

He is a reliable worker but, he says, he is fed up. He would like to retire and go home to live. He talks enthusiastically about the week-end he is having at home soon and about the Chadwick fête in a couple of weeks.

'It's my brain,' he said by way of explanation over lunch when he was trying to remember something. He gave his head an irritated tap. You find yourself wondering if these young men and women are aware that they are mentally handicapped and what it means. Some of them are, Mrs G says. At the conference she attended, where they talked about marriage and the mentally handicapped, one man had explained that he could not marry because he could not support a wife on £2 a week and another had reasoned that it was not possible because he was mentally handicapped and therefore incapable of living alone without supervision. That was the difference in levels of understanding.

'One of our boys insists that he is only here because he has had a nervous breakdown. He did have a breakdown, but one reason for it was him trying to cope with the strain of a simple job in the outside world. On the surface he seems a borderline case, but when you get to know him, there are many simple little tasks he cannot do.'

11.30 a.m.

A group arrive back in the farmyard from the fields, on a trailer attached to a tractor. The driver, M, is a farm instructor. He was in similar work previously, but not with the mentally handicapped. He admits he has had to get used to some pretty frustrating days, when his workforce is uncooperative and nothing gets done.

The philosophy of the Home is that this does not matter. A surprise, this, as the public idea of these Homes is that they try very hard to be self-supporting.

'The happiness of the residents is the main concern,' a spokesman for the organization pointed out. 'Being a business must never get in the way of that. We have had to lose some managers because they were too efficient. They got too involved in making the places pay.'

It must be hard not to, if you are efficient by nature. M lives out, as do all the instructors. Only houseparents live in. That, M says, requires dedication, which he does not possess. He needs his daily breaks. He told me a story about a dainty little housemother, who was thrown by her long hair across the room by a jealous resident who had a crush on her husband.

Neither the husband, also a member of the care staff, nor the housemother, who was hurt and shaken, showed any sign of anger towards the girl. 'He helped her up. She went outside the door to catch her breath for a minute and they both carried on as if nothing had happened. That is dedication to the job.'

It also shows that life at Chadwick House is not always as calm and ordered as it appears.

There are twenty people on the staff. Mr and Mrs G, a part-time administrator, a farm instructor, a gardening instructor, two craft teachers (young women who left teachers' training college with the mid-Seventies bulge and could not find conventional jobs), ten care staff, three domestics and a cook.

For thirty-one able-bodied people, who do some of the work themselves, it sounds plenty. But, like everywhere else, they feel short-staffed. There are often only two care people on at a time, Mr G says, and it is not enough.

They look, they say, for people who are qualified (though in what is not mentioned!) and 'people to whom it is not just a job'. There is in-service training for staff spread over sixteen weeks. 'Different people come to speak – a psychiatrist, an expert in drama therapy, someone in residential work and so on.'

12.45 p.m. – The Craft Room

There are two workshops for crafts: one is a hut, the other a farm outbuilding, with a teacher running each. But in summer, when I was there, there were only enough enthusiasts to fill the hut, none of them involved in anything very ambitious.

Four girls are sewing teddy bear shapes by hand. One of the teachers does some finishing off on the electric sewing-machine. They are getting a hand-operated one she says, which some of the girls will be able to manage. The teachers are working hard at making things like cute cotton purses on strings, for the fête. A lot of stuff is provided by parents' and Friends' groups and they man the stalls, helped by the more able residents.

There are two boys in the craft room. Ian, who would, I think, be described as a non-contributor, is scribbling on a piece of paper. ('We move him around to give him some variety,' Mrs G explained) and Harry, who returns with the swimming party.

Harry is a tall, curly-haired eighteen-year-old, with the sort of face you might expect to see smiling down from a teenage girl's poster collection. He is gentle, refined and polite to excess. His refinement does not necessarily make him popular. The other boys who share his room do not share his passion for classical music and he has to take his records down to the kitchen to play them.

He is one of the most able talkers in the Home, with a good memory and the ability to put his coherent thoughts into equally coherent words. There is, however, the weird feeling of listening to a carefully programmed computer. Mrs G insists that his opinions are his own. He talked at the conference and will repeat every word at the drop of a hat or deliver any other speech the occasion calls for.

Harry likes craftwork. 'Here, boys do not have to do one job and girls another, like in some places,' he said. 'You can do what you like. I think that is good.'

1 p.m.

Lunch is light in summer, Mrs G has explained, because dinner is the main meal. The residents sit at long tables for up to eight people in a dining-room adjoining the big, well-equipped kitchen. They have their own regular place at table and staff eat with them.

May, the cook, is in charge of the kitchen, with helpers from among the residents. Breakfast is at 8 a.m. (8 to 10 on Saturday and Sunday). There is a coffee break at 10.30, lunch at 1 p.m. and work finishes at 4.30 with time to get washed and changed for dinner at 6 p.m.

Lunch is on the table when everyone goes in. A tiny salad – basically an egg and a few lettuce leaves, with rolls and butter. At Tom's table, where I sit, there is much discussion of sharing out of spare rolls. One boy with a lovely cheeky grin ('and a very devious nature,' Mrs G added) gets through four apart from his own. There is some weak tea to follow. Altogether not too filling for open-air appetites. The second time I had lunch there – it is a hospitable place – there was someone from head office present and the meal was grander. It could have been coincidence.

Then, the after-dinner speeches, thanking the guest – me – for coming. Three of the more vocal residents say their pieces, approaching Mr G at the top of a table first for permission. There is great applause from the rest of the room for their efforts. It is a regular procedure with visitors. Hospitable, but a little alarming. It makes you feel a bit like the Queen, and must go down a treat with fund-raising groups and more official callers.

5 p.m.

Some of the residents have washed and changed already and are divided between the two lounges: one for noisy pursuits, mostly playing records; the other the quiet room for television-watching.

A few people are still upstairs, washing or bathing. The majority can manage alone and simply come and go as they please about the house. A few need assistance or encouragement. S, a young house-mother, hurries about between bathroom and the newly built laundry, where machines are going, virtually every waking hour. There are shelves and pigeon-holes for each resident's clothes and it is another area where residents work.

The television room has plenty of armchairs lining the walls and a suite plus coffee table at the furthest end. Mr and Mrs G take visitors in here for coffee, and now a boy and girl sit there, arms round each other, ignoring the rest.

Inevitably the question of sexual relationships crops up. Mrs G is aware of the possibilities. She and the staff are keeping a low profile but monitoring certain situations, she says. They know what is going on and so far have seen no reason to put any girl on the pill.

Half-a-dozen people are crowded around the set, watching children's programmes. There is some squabbling from those behind who cannot see and one young man dressed like a rising executive, with a sheaf of papers in his hand, arrives complaining bitterly that someone has been unkind to him.

Judy, who was out in the fields in jeans and wellies, is wearing a many-toned dress and some rather amateurishly applied lipstick and eye shadow. The residents wear their own clothes, bought by parents, but if parents fall behind with provision, they are bought from Home funds. Judy wonders where her boyfriend is and Tom, somewhat alarmingly, informs her that he has fallen asleep in the bath.

Tom is joined by his friend Donald, in his late twenties with a blond moustache and green army-style sweater with shoulder patches. This is the man who had a nervous breakdown, another single-roomer. 'I'm Donald, Don to my friends,' he introduces himself, taking the initiative with a firm hand-shake. As he takes his hand away, you realize it is shaking. Such is the effort that goes into his apparent normality.

The room fills up gradually. Two male care assistants join the crowd. Until then there has been no supervision. A loud male resident persists in standing in front of the television, talking and blocking everyone's view. One of the care assistants leans forward and gives him a light kick, which understandably makes him even noisier.

6 p.m. Dinner

Everyone processes through the 'noisy' lounge, into the dining-room. It is spaghetti bolognaise tonight, as I have been told a dozen times. It turns out to be flavourless mince, with practically no sauce, followed by jelly and cream.

R, one of the care staff – housefather doesn't seem to fit – at my table, is young, single and started his career in advertising. He got dispirited with the money-grubbing, wanted to do something useful. This is not the first Home for the mentally handicapped he has worked in, but it is, he says, 'the most natural'.

'The residents are allowed to do things for themselves, instead of being told or having it all done for them.'

6.30 p.m.

Dinner over, the kitchen is packed with helpers. There is a dish-washer, but it is not considered very efficient. May washes up and a couple of girls dry. Other residents come in to look, deliver a message or pass through – but stop to talk. It is hard to know how many have a purpose but nobody is sent away.

May is a local widow, warm and friendly, as much a social worker/mother-figure as a cook. She took the job when her husband died and has become completely involved with it, going away on their seaside holiday, welcoming them into the kitchen to solve problems.

Harry brings his records down and plays them to her, but tonight he has only come to talk – about freedom. It was his topic at the conference, his belief that he and other residents should have more freedom to come and go as they please. Mr G doesn't mind him saying what he thinks, he adds quickly.

He talks slowly and clearly. He can write and read, on the level of a young child. His official label was autistic and he spent several years at a boarding-school before coming to Chadwick. Not that Harry is in any way rejected. His mother sat before the PSA meeting holding his hand and he goes home for occasional weekends. His younger, normal brother goes to boarding-school, too. It is that kind of busy, professional family.

'I think a lot of parents find it hard to part with their teenagers,' Mrs G reasons, 'but if they don't take a place now, there won't be one when they are older.'

Where would Harry go if he had this freedom? To the pub, he said. Alone. There are not many places to go near Chadwick House. Even the village shop is shut when work is over, so pocket money can only be spent on Saturdays. Occasionally one or two will go with a staff member to the local pub and on most evenings the more energetic residents ride around the grounds on their bikes, or down the road if there is a staff member to go with them. Nobody, surprisingly, takes it into his or her head, simply to wander off alone. There are no locked gates, no one dogging their heels.

Birthday girls and boys have the choice of a trip to the pub with a few friends or a disco session in the lounge. There had been a disco the night before and the girl celebrating had cut short a trip home to get back in time. She was still walking around with the decorative band from her cake pinned round her head.

7.30 p.m.

The kitchen has been cleared of people, expect for May, Harry and S, the housemother, pausing for a cup of tea. She is a pretty girl who used to be a ground hostess at an airport until she met and married a male nurse. He is now one of three male care assistants at Chadwick and they have a flat in the house.

Yes, it is inconvenient, sometimes, living in, she agrees. Even if you are off duty, your door is conveniently close when problems crop up. And of course there are no real career prospects working in a small Home, nor high wages, but if you wanted those things you wouldn't take the job. She wanted, she says, to help people, while she is young and healthy and free to – and they get a lot back from the residents.

Care staff work shifts, from 7 a.m. till 3 p.m. and from 2 till 10 p.m, with two days off a week. They take turns going round to check twice during the night – otherwise there are no night staff. During the week, most residents get to bed around 9 p.m. At weekends, residents and houseparents often sit up to watch the late movie on television.

While S talks, one of the boys – a mongol and no taller than she –

hangs on to her arm, his head against her shoulder. Later, in the lounge, he sits at her feet, watching television, while her good-looking husband sits beside her. It is inevitable that some of the residents become attached to individuals, and essential that they should neither reject nor show favouritism, they say.

Harry, who seems to identify almost exclusively with staff rather than residents, which can be a lonely occupation, said he didn't have a girlfriend at the Home. At his previous place, he used to prefer the housemothers. He walks out to my car with me. Most of the residents are in one or other of the lounges. Harry is not planning to join them. He is going up to his room to write letters. There are quarrels in his room sometimes, he says, but he does not believe in quarrelling: it is a waste of time – you have to live together. He is full of such homilies.

Would he prefer to live at home? 'I expect I would get bored after a while,' he says carefully. Suddenly he spots the heading on a leaflet I am holding about the Home. 'It says this is a place for children,' he says indignantly. 'Whoever wrote that made a mistake. There are no children here. We are all adults.'

Conclusions

Whether or not the basic concept of Chadwick and the other Homes like it is your cup of tea, you've got to admit the progress from parents' project to highly professional organization has been phenomenal.

The mother of the first child into the first Home, puts it down simply to 'dedication'. 'We were all willing to take risks, mortgage ourselves up to the hilt to ensure security for our children.'

There is more to it than that. The pioneers were families with enough cash between them to get the project off the ground. Many families, however dedicated, could not have laid hands on a couple of thousand pounds. They were people who, though not professionally involved in the field of mental handicap, were informed. They knew where to go looking for further information and help. Though they rely a lot on charity, the Homes depended almost entirely for support on the parents, in the early days. They, in turn, seem to have had an uncanny knack of knowing exactly when to hand over to paid professionals.

In the beginning there were six families, with children attending the same boarding-school and due to leave when they reached sixteen. A far-sighted head teacher called a parents' meeting and put it to them that their children would soon be returning home or to institutional care and would, either way, probably regress without mental stimulation. The alternative, he pointed out, was to open a Home themselves – a place that would give them as warm a home life and as stimulating an atmosphere as their school had.

A teacher at the school agreed to be the first resident manager if the scheme could be got off the ground. The parents, all from the immediate area, formed a committee.

The first chairman, Mr T remembers: 'We used to hold meetings in my front room, working out the legal aspects, getting registered as a charity, finding a name and deciding what, exactly, we were looking for. We all knew it was a good idea, but we didn't know much else. We wanted to base the Home on agriculture, but initially we were looking at 200-acre farms. It was completely unrealistic.'

Gradually it became clear that their £11,000 would not stretch to a full-scale self-supporting village. The money had come from the parents themselves, including £6,000 from one family. Seven hundred pounds went immediately on purchasing the first old Manor House in thirteen acres – the rest on doing it up and equipping it in a small way.

It was furnished on a shoe-string, a second-hand string at that. Mrs C remembers getting a friend with a lorry to go from door to door begging old furniture.

They made, they admit, a few mistakes – expecting too much of the residents, for a start. Cattle proved an extravagant disaster. The residents could not cope with them. Pigs, poultry and horticulture were a big success – and still are.

'We gave them plenty to do outside,' Mr T said, 'but it cannot be described as a village community. They are not self-contained and we did not want them to be. In some Homes, residents go out to simple jobs locally. I would call them sheltered communities.'

Another early shock was the rapid turnover of residential staff. They have come to accept that this happens everywhere, but that one way round it, particularly with managers, was to pay a competetive salary.

Mr T: 'We started off thinking that dedicated people would find their way to us however little we paid. It was a mistake. When you think of it, we are almost asking the impossible of our managers. They have to be able to talk to parents, management and staff, bring out the best in the residents – deal with masses of paperwork. We have to have complete confidence in them as substitute parents for our children.'

Has the Trust evolved as the early pioneers foresaw? Yes, Mr T says, except that it has grown larger and faster, which is all to the good.

'Initially we just wanted security for life for our children – a second home. The beauty of this is that it is parent-orientated. Parents go in any time to see the child, take him out, have him home for weekends whenever they want.'

Parent power, however, is less obtrusive now than it was. There has been a gradual delegating of the running to professionals.

Ten years ago a general manager was appointed and the relevant office staff. Four years ago an appeals officer joined them to encourage existing Friends groups, instigate many others and rally the help of the usual fund-raising groups from Girl Guides to Rotarians.

Major Trust decisions are mulled over by the Council – which consists of eighteen people, sixteen of them parents. Above them is an Executive Council and parents are represented here, too. Mr T is adamant that he and other parents still have a strong voice.

Do they, I wondered, ever take residents whose parents cannot contribute at all financially?

'We have done,' he said, 'but obviously we could not take too many because we need the support.'

'There is no means test, but parents are interviewed about finances and I think all of them give fairly, what they can afford. Many people leave a sizeable amount in their wills for their children's future upkeep and we do expect parents to make some arrangement of this kind.'

You cannot, on the other hand, buy a place. All prospective residents are given a six-month trial. Irrespective of financial arrangements, if they do not fit in or disrupt the rest, they have to go.

Chadwick is élitist, middle-class, conservative, very British. It is a strange combination of old ideas, new ideas and positively ancient ideas reincarnated.

In line with current thinking, jobs are more varied and stretching than the average Adult Training Centre workshop. But it turns its back on modern notions of community living. There are no neighbours, at least not close enough for a chat over the garden fence without a loud-hailer. They do not go out to work, hence another source of outside contact is removed.

The residents are cushioned – though living in groups of this size brings its own stress – and though they go out and visitors come in, some seem to feel the isolation. It shows in their excitement at the sight of visitors.

Some could not easily function except under supervision. But what of gregarious people like Tom? The superficially normal who strive to be more so, like Donald? The practical and capable, like Neil, and the confident and articulate like Harry? They could live in a Group Home, in virtually any community and lead lives that are nearly normal. Should they be encouraged to do so?

The forward-looking professionals would say yes. The parents say no . . . and this is one place where parents' feelings count. I took two mothers of handicapped adult daughters with me on one visit. They loved Chadwick House. It was perfection. The setting, the brightness and cleanliness of the house, the beauty of the gardens and fields were vital factors in their approval. So was the charm of the people who run it and the politeness and after-dinner speeches of the residents.

'Even if our daughters will never live here,' said one mother (one girl is too handicapped, the other past the upper age limit), 'it warms your heart to think that people have built something so perfect. Maybe the authorities will copy it.'

Maybe they will, but it is doubtful. They could learn a lot, especially about giving parents what they want – and, hopefully what their children want, too. Statutory providers, though, do not have the luxury of being able to choose residents and their parents. Inevitably there would be difficult and more handicapped residents and disinterested families who drifted apart. Inevitably it would be a different place.

THE VILLAGE – ANOTHER VARIATION ON THE THEME

Sheldon Village is just what it says – a single street, a cluster of bungalows, a few offices, a recreation hall, some workshops to provide cottage industry employment for the villagers – all mentally handicapped. There are thirty acres of land, some of it given over to horticulture.

Like any village, it is isolated but, unlike the villages of old, there is no corner shop, no pub, no village post-office or church. In short, no natural spots for easy socializing and community life.

Sheldon, then, is not your natural-grown community, but more of the hot-house variety, forced up over a few years. To quote the manager, until 1973 the whole site was 'just a green field'.

It was the second of five villages set up by this voluntary organization – this particular village with much financial help from a parent, who is now a highly motivated, unpaid fund-raiser for the organization.

The living accommodation – 'cottages' with twelve separate single rooms attached – is good, but the village as a whole has a bleak, naked, newborn look. Perhaps time will help there. The charity's literature concedes that villages built around an existing old house and its grounds are the ideal. It also regards nine to twelve individuals of mixed sex as the right number for any living unit – not so small that individuals can get on each other's nerves, not big enough to be institutional.

It is, of course, a million miles from community care. Only a little less, it seems, from the nearest town! It is isolated, with public transport none too good. Perhaps this would not be a major problem if all the facilities were provided on the campus. With only the all-purpose recreation hall/dining-room, staging twice-weekly events, it matters.

Nevertheless, the village has many things going for it. The manager says they insist on purposeful work for the forty villagers – and the carpenters among them were making some magnificent, Galt-style wooden toys, kitchen utensils, shelves and even beds. Others were printing, some packing and a group of women made soft toys and rugs. They take on no contract work and the place does not aim to be anywhere near self-sufficient, but the products sell easily at village events and through a mail-order catalogue.

Unlike Chadwick – and more practically – villagers are not allowed total freedom of choice as to which job they do. Those with a particular interest and ability – like the mongol boy on the printing press printing Christmas cards, and the autistic young man making wooden toys – are encouraged to specialize.

'Others will always be generalists,' Mr H, the manager explained. So residents help around the village – in the kitchens, the laundry, the grounds, the gardens (they grow all their own fruit and vegetables), with new building projects. There is no farming here, though other villages go in for it in a big way.

Each cottage has a large common lounge and kitchen, where breakfast and supper are cooked. There are eighteen people on the payroll. Two resident care assistants live in each cottage in their own flat, but only one is on duty at a time – a very low staff ratio, only feasible, presumably, because the villagers are high-grade, fit young people.

Even so, Mr H estimates that one-fifth are non-productive in the sense of contributing nothing workwise to the village, and two residents are positively counter-productive.

IQ, he says, is not a factor taken greatly into account for entry. Being able-bodied and sociable are the two first essentials.

Willingness on the part of the prospective villager's Local Authority to pay his or her fees is another vital point. If not, they cannot be considered. Parents are not asked to contribute, though several involve themselves in fund-raising. It is not – again, differently from Chadwick – a consideration for entry.

Surprisingly, there is not an endlessly long waiting list or agonizing over the numbers who have to be turned away. When everything is taken into account, they tend, Mr H thinks, to be self-selecting. Fees are £68 a week – not wildly expensive when you consider that no extra Adult Training Centre charge will be needed, as there is at an ordinary residential unit where people go out to sheltered work during the day. The villager's own Social Security allowances – around £20 – make up part of the fee. They keep only £3.80 for personal spending.

Fees match running costs exactly. Capital funds still come by way of donations and fund-raising. There is a central office for the group of villages, with one paid publicist/fund-raiser. They do not find they have to mount big campaigns. The cash-flow from this quarter is reassuringly regular and comes often 'from the personal touch'. There are small, local fund-raising groups, but not on the scale of for instance, Chadwick's Friends.

Staff from the deputy manager down are not required to have any 'paper qualifications'. Care staff are often young people waiting to go to university or to train for jobs in the field of mental handicap.

Mr H: 'I'd rather have a vivacious, intelligent, lively person for a year than a dull, unimaginative one who would stay for ten. So would the villagers. They don't resent one person leaving as long as they like the next. It is a mistake, in my opinion, to think their feelings are as deep as that. They get over people going very quickly, even parents dying. They are everybody's friend, like children.

'People often come to work in the village through friends. Unions are resented. 'We try to pay a bit more so that we can keep unionism out.'

Ultimate decisions for all five villages are the prerogative of a board of directors, including some parents who also happen to be businessmen with useful skills. Beneath them is an executive committee for day-to-day running. There is a parent on this but, all-in-all, parents are not heavily represented. Each village manager has a lot of autonomy.

It is perhaps not fair to keep comparing the village with Chadwick, but their similarities make it tempting. I found it a much more hard-headed place, superficially anyway. My visit was briefer and I did not get to know individuals. The villagers seemed more self-contained, less dependent on staff, and the jobs – at least those of the 'specialists' – were more demanding and presumably more satisfying.

There was a noticeable difference of attitudes. The feeling, in the village, for example, that we over-estimate the attachments of mentally handicapped people towards staff and towards each other. 'We've only had one sexual relationship here over the years. We don't encourage it. There is too much talk about the sexual feelings of the mentally handicapped lately – mainly by people who don't know them. It is just something that has become fashionable.'

And the cussed question of what will happen when the present villagers are no longer young and able-bodied. There are no definite plans. There is talk of a retirement cottage, a nursing home elsewhere; the firm feeling that they will not be able to continue living in the village – their home, remember – if they become 'physically handicapped, senile or incontinent'.

Practical commonsense, or devaluing of people's feelings? It depends on how you look at it. 'We are not a nursing organization,' Mr H. says. True – but parents who had given a sigh of relief convinced they had found their child a home for life would have trouble seeing it so objectively.

Sheldon Village is, simply and unsentimentally, a place for the able-bodied, reasonably capable mentally handicapped to live and work in a sheltered environment. They would not claim to cater for anything but a narrow section of the population.

A staff member who was just leaving wrote an article for the newsletter which criticized the practice in the village of sending residents to bed at 9.30. It was pointed out that this happened only with the less able who needed supervision, but nevertheless it was printed.

Mr H says that what they have built at Sheldon is exactly what he and the other pioneers envisaged when faced with the green field and the brief to build the ideal home for a group of mentally handicapped people.

He has perfect confidence that the village way is the right way and, increasingly, more and more people are beginning to agree.

HINDLEY HOME – BUILT BY A LOCAL SOCIETY

Hindley Home is another example of parents doing it their way. It is a three-storey, purpose-built residential unit for over-sixteens, paid for and run by a local society for the mentally handicapped with 500 members – only sixty of them 'working members', according to the chairman.

The Home was built two years ago out of the proceeds of an appeal lasting five years. It cost £70,000. Nearly ten years before that, the society had built Hindley House, an all-purpose hall and meeting-place for members. Now the two stand side-by-side. The residents of the Home can attend clubs, evening classes and socials held in the hall, with outside members.

A charge is made to Local Authorities for each resident placed. The whole campus, as the society headquarters, generates a startling annual turnover of £75,000 and is administered by non-professionals, officers of the society . . . 'though of course we call in the professionals – solicitors, accountants, architects – when we need them,' said the chairman.

In practice, talk of running the place brings you inevitably to Mr R, the chairman – one of those human dynamos you occasionally get out front in such organizations.

He has just retired from a job in management and spends much of his day in a small office in the Home, doing an administrator's job. He does not call it that, though, and is scornful of similar Homes taking on paid, professional administrators. 'What you need in charge of a place like this, is someone efficient, who can run it as a business, but has heart,' he says, hand clamped appropriately to bosom.

Mr H's whole family is involved. Introducing a daughter who runs a club in the hall, he pointed out: 'You have to think of the future and get young people involved. It has to carry on when I'm not here.' His wife is one of a selection committee of three (with a doctor and a teacher) which accepts or rejects applicants. They have turned down three in three years for the usual reason – that they were incontrollable and wrecked the place.

Mr H has a mentally handicapped adult son, living at home. He wants him eventually to come to the Home when and if the family cannot cope any more – as indeed do most of the parents who were involved in the project, but usually only when they die.

That creates problems. It will not be possible to always have a place vacant at the right moment. 'The members will do anything to help', said Mr H, 'but the one thing they won't do for me is die to order.'

He keeps places vacant. There are only ten residents in the actual Home, with five sleeping in a nearby Council house, as a sort of annexe. When the housemother and her family move out of their flat on the top floor and into a Council house backing on the complex, there will be eight more places.

It still isn't enough, so Mr H plans to rent more Council accommodation – they are in the middle of a Council estate in a small town – for abler residents, and also buy one or two houses around as they become available. The society is looking out for its first purchase at the moment. All with an eye to more places as they are needed – quite soon, he feels, with many of the involved members getting old.

He's been accused of empire-building, he says wryly, but cannot think of a more worthwhile cause for which to build empires. Fund-raising is apparently no problem. He talks to local schools, clubs and any other organization which will listen; rallies members to keep up the society's efforts – and they always manage to keep afloat. There has to be a substantial sum in the kitty always to tide them over because Local Authorities can be late paying.

Society members have some say in how the Home should be built and run, but not all that much. Nor it seems, do they want to.

'You have to be a bit of a dictator,' said Mr H. Clearly he enjoys the role. How did he decide what was needed? By asking himself if that facility would suit his handicapped son. If the answer was yes, then it would suit most of the other residents too.

He is a great believer in parents knowing best where the mentally handicapped are concerned. Little incidents would appear to prove him right. Crash doors in case of fire, for example. Professionals, he says, have always assumed the mentally handicapped could open the doors themselves. Mr H doubted it, checked it out – and found they could not. An alternative system of opening them from the outside had to be fitted.

The Home has a lot in common – in size, function, position and age and ability of residents – with Local Authority hostels. Again, 'hostel' has become one of those mental handicap terms that can be interpreted loosely – but it is a 'good' word, smacking of freedom, small numbers and community living for the handicapped.

Mr H and his staff will not have it used in connection with their Home, however. He says: 'We went to great lengths to make this a real home, a family unit. We do not intend it to turn into a glorified mini-institution, with staff clocking on and off like a factory, as has happened in some hostels.'

It is a surprisingly active organization. Societies of this kind have an unfortunate tendency to centre around a few, often ageing, stalwart parents and get very stuck in the mud. Mr H and his band are forward-looking, particularly where the Home residents are concerned. Evening classes have just been started in the hall, to teach 'survival skills', like how to make a cup of tea and toast. There is a weekly swimming class – with pupils who have done well enough to enter a gala. Three teachers run a morning class in the hall, teaching 'ineducable' adults to read and write – with great success. Home residents have the advantage of all the society's clubs and facilities on the doorstep. A big advantage. They cannot be isolated.

The Home has recently acquired its own band of friends, none of them parents or society members, but all local people who plan to take a continuing interest in the residents. It is all part of the plan to have someone to visit and help with fund-raising when parents are no longer here – as, indeed, has already happened with some of the present residents.

The Friends visit on Sunday and each individual or couple takes a special interest in one resident, taking him or her for a walk or even home to tea. Not everyone is fixed up with a Friend yet. Inevitably there are some difficult customers among the residents; and in any case, the Friends split naturally into two groups – those who wanted to mix with the mentally handicapped, and those who wanted to raise funds but gave individuals a wide berth.

The Home itself is neat and new, with its single and twin-bedded rooms done out in matching shades. Clinically so, one member of staff from another Home based in an old house commented, intimating it would always have an institutional air. I don't think it matters. The quality of life depends on deeper things than how the bricks are arranged.

Friday 5.30 p.m.

The residents are arriving home from the Adult Training Centre. A few are already in or have been here all day due to minor ailments. They come in – as does everyone except VIPS – through the kitchen door and then move about as they please. To one of the two lounges or, as most do, hang around the kitchen/dining area, waiting for tea.

The kitchen/dining-room is one long building with no division bar a waist-high counter. The kitchen is well equipped and well laid out with plenty of space. Clever, too: there are *two* of the appliances most likely to give trouble due to breakdown or strikes – a gas *and* an electric cooker, two fridges, two freezers, two vacuum cleaners.

This was one of the tricks the committee picked up from visits to other residential places in the planning stage. Barring very bad luck, they are covered for all eventualities.

The kitchen area is furnished with big pine tables and a matching pine sideboard. One of the care assistants is cooking the evening meal – fried sausages and tomato, bread and butter, tea, and with a banana or orange to follow. They have their main meal at midday at work. Later, at 8.30, there is a hot drink and a piece of cake, for anyone who is in.

The place never seems crowded or even full, because there is a lot of space, and the fifteen residents is a figure well below full complement. Only half-a-dozen people sit down at the table at this sitting. The other tables are empty. The rest of the residents will be served as they come in. It is a flexible system. It has to be. Transport to and from the Adult Training Centre can be unpredictable. Staff complain that, because it is a Home, the Department seem to think it doesn't matter if transport is late or even fails to turn up some evenings.

They are a surprisingly old group of people at the table, predominantly middle-aged. Most have come from hospitals, a few straight from home. Bob, a middle-aged mongol, is one of these. He was looked after all his life by a devoted mother who took care of his every whim. She died and he found himself in the Home and under the wing of another 'mother'.

Doreen, his mother-figure substitute, is actually a few years younger than Bob. She is forty, looks and (in patches anyway) sounds normal, and came here from a hospital. She doesn't, she emphasizes, want to go back to the hospital ('They made me work hard there.')

In fact, immediately prior to her transfer to the Home, she was living out in digs and only going into the hospital workshop during the day. One reason for moving her here is the extra supervision. Doreen was apparently taking advantage of her freedom to a worrying degree.

She has, her records say, a passion for lame ducks. In Bob, she has found one. He almost sits on her lap throughout tea. When a wasp buzzes around, he grabs hold of her arm and she has to shoo it away. Later in the evening, he is to be found in the television room, asleep with his head on her shoulder.

This total reliance of Bob's used to worry the staff, but not half as much as Doreen's other relationship – with Nigel. Nigel makes up the final third of what the staff call the terrible trio. His feelings for Doreen, however, are not those of an adopted son, but definitely sexual.

'It doesn't seem to go beyond wandering hands,' said the assistant housemother, Judy. 'All the same, it can be embarrassing. I suggest you knock before going into the television room. *I* wish he wouldn't do it in church!

'It is a problem, the whole thing. The two men follow Doreen everywhere. If she is in the loo, you will find them waiting outside. She teases them and plays them off against each other. She is a very powerful lady. We have tried separating the three of them, but Bob gets distressed and Nigel becomes very physical and aggressive.'

It is a problem that Mr H, chairman of the local society that built and runs the Home and their part-time administrator, does not acknowledge. Or if he does, he was not sharing it with me.

'We don't get sexual situations occurring,' he said. 'What we wanted to build here was a family unit and that's how the residents see themselves: fifteen members of a family. You get quarrels and disagreements – you would with fifteen normal adults living together – but it is a family with a Mum at the head of it.'

'Mum' is Mrs S, the housemother who lives with her husband and three children in a flat on the second floor. Her husband 'helps out with driving, shaving, things like that' but follows his own occupation.

The first time I saw Mrs S, she was giving a talk on being a housemother, and stressing – uncomfortably I felt – the aspect of being 'Mum' to all the residents. They all call her that, she said. A few do – which sounds ridiculous coming from the older ones – but in practice most of them in my hearing referred to her as Mrs S. That is no detraction from her competence, rather the reverse. The majority of the residents may be fond of her and rely on her, but they must be aware of having had a mother and feel past the stage for adopting a new one. It is a little condescending.

Doreen is one of the people who does call her Mum – to her face but not when talking about her. 'Jean [a new resident, rather disturbed and unsociable] hit me in the face, Mum,' she said over tea, near to tears. 'She did, hit me here. Why did she do it, Mum?'

Jean meanwhile had left the table and was on her way upstairs. She spends all her time in her room. Mrs S suggests Doreen should stand up for herself and hit back. Later, another member of staff confronted with the same bit of news tells her this is precisely what she must not do. Doreen looks confused. The housemother does punish wrongdoers, mainly those who indulge in bad language, by withdrawal of privileges – no Gateway Club or no television.

Doreen chats throughout the meal – about the education programme she is doing at the Centre: 'I can write my name now and I can make a cup of tea. I can make one for Mrs S'. She works in the kitchen at the Centre, a privileged position, and, she says proudly, gets a bonus.

None of them will get rich on their 'take-home pay' from the Centre. It varies from 50p. to £1.50. They give it to the housemother and get back £2 pocket money as and when they ask for it. Mostly it is spent on records, tapes for cassettes (most of them seem to have one or other in their rooms), writing paper, make-up for the few girls who use a little lipstick and face cream, and drinks if they go out with a member of staff to the local pub in the evening. One of Mr H's hopes for the future is a sheltered workshop on the site, with no pressure to be totally self-supporting, but paying a real wage.

Nothing conventional. He is toying with the idea of a car wash or a laundry.

Officially each resident has to have £3.50 pocket money each week but some is saved for holidays (this year they went to Blackpool) and outings. They go out with the Home staff, with the league of friends and with the Gateway Club for the mentally handicapped which holds weekly meetings in the hall adjoining the Home. There is an impressive list of pantomimes and shows in the nearby city theatres listed for visiting over the next couple of months.

Tea over, Mrs S helps one of the men with shaving (there is a razor power-point in the kitchen), gives the youngest boy, eighteen-year-old Larry, the batteries she has bought for him and then goes upstairs. She is not officially on duty, but living over the shop has its problems.

'Even when she is on holiday, she has to keep popping in for emergencies,' one of the staff said. As mentioned at the beginning of this chapter, there are plans to use a recently acquired Council house nearby for the housemother and her family and turn her flat into accommodation for eight.

The staff consist of Mrs S, with a deputy housemother who is there when Mrs S is off-duty and who sleeps in a couple of nights a week. There are two care assistants and eight auxiliary workers – local women who give a hand with everything.

They are not paid rates competitive with Local Authority hostels and more is expected of them. 'More flexibility' is how Mr H describes it. 'If one of the women who comes in to do domestic work is asked to help one of the residents bath, she doesn't say it is not her job. If Mrs S is going into town and there is an emergency, she will come back, cancel her plans and take over.'

The staff themselves are well aware of their 'unequal' status and insist they do not mind. 'Money doesn't bother me, nor the hours, as long as I am happy in the job,' said Mrs S, who is a trained nurse and has worked in Local Authority children's homes.

6.30 p.m.

Doreen is in the television lounge – one of two adjoining lounges opening off the dining-room. Bob sits beside her, a rug covering their knees, his head on her shoulder, a ring she gave him on his finger.

He is tired, she says, giving him a squeeze. She will put him to bed after a while. He cannot stay up till 9.30 or 10.0 p.m. like the others.

Nigel sits at her feet, glaring at me for distracting her, glaring at Bob who is getting so much attention. At one point Bob wakes up sufficiently to lean forward and playfully pretend to strangle Nigel. Doreen suddenly bursts into tears and is comforted and patted by both men. Her sister has not written to her, she says. She was expecting a letter. In fact, the housemother explained, the sister – her only family connection – calls about once a year, but Doreen talks of her and her niece continually. Her mother drowned herself, Doreen goes on to sob and she found her. 'She was wearing my new shoes. There was water in her eyes.'

It is an incongruous scene. The trio are completely self-absorbed. The other four women watching television ignore them. Mostly they ignore each other, too. Doreen sleeps out of the Home at night. She and four other women have been moved – for sleeping purposes anyway – to a smartly modernized Council house within sight of the Home.

The Council has rented it to them as a group dwelling for the most able, a half-way house to break them into the idea of living without supervision. At the moment, though, it is a home in name only – rather a waste. The women sleep there – with a night care assistant sleeping downstairs – but arrive for breakfast at the main Home at around 8.0 a.m. and do not go back again till 9.30 p.m.

They are not responsible for housework, nor do they attempt to get their meals or – apart from one girl – deal with their own laundry, though the house is well-equipped with domestic appliances.

There is no training programme to encourage independent living, although residents are encouraged to help with chores at the Home: washing up, sweeping outside, emptying bins. Only those who are interested do it. I didn't, for instance, ever see Doreen helping in the kitchen despite her ability. She says, though, that she would like to have a television in the house, cook her own meals and generally live there. At the moment it would be beyond her. What skills she is picking up for future use come mainly from the Adult Training Centre.

The second lounge is larger, nicely carpeted, with the same arrangement of new chairs set out around three of the four walls. This layout of the furniture immediately screams institution, but there is nothing you can do about it when you have to provide seating for so many people. There are two people at one end of the room, a man and a woman, sitting several seats apart, and the two youngest boys at the other end, beside a record player.

Larry is playing his records, bringing each one right up to his nose to peer at it before deciding to put it on the player or discard it. A little earlier he had been in the kitchen, helping the assistant housemother, Judy, to make jelly, looking at each packet with the same concentration. He seems, despite his limited sight, much more lively and capable than most of the other residents.

'I know you shouldn't have favourites,' Judy said, as he gave her a hug, 'but he's mine.'

7.30 p.m.

Judy is making scones and sausage-rolls in the kitchen, managing despite the 'help' of an eighteen-year-old who arrived a few days before – and who I believed, till told otherwise, to be one of the helpers. The girl picks up bits of pastry and rolls them into a ball, makes requests for goldfish to keep in her room, then a rabbit and a cat. Fortunately or unfortunately, pets are not allowed.

One of the men, in his twenties, who is obsessively concerned about another resident not liking the Home, hovers around the table, too. In the small laundry room off the kitchen one woman resident is doing the ironing, aided – verbally at least – by two friends.

All three are very sociable and talkative, but difficult to understand. The ironer lived alone with her elderly mother, looked after her, and did all the housework until the old lady died. Besides Judy, there is one general helper on duty and she is washing up, assisted by one of the female residents, who dries and puts away cutlery, as well as doing her favourite job – always kept for her – of squeezing out tea-bags.

Later on, this helper goes upstairs at the request of one of the older residents, to give her a hand with having a bath. There are two very 'posh' bathrooms – one for men, one for women – plus showers. Baths are taken twice a week on rota, but it is flexible. Judy had been too busy to do any rota baths tonight, but this lady had asked and wasn't discouraged.

Judy worked hard at her baking all evening – and did not, in two hours, go into the lounges to speak to the residents. So much for

Mr H's insistence that nearly all domestic tasks are taken from housemothers to leave them time to be with the residents, giving individual attention.

'If she spent just fifteen minutes with each one, that's nearly four hours. I'd be hard put to itemize what a Mum does at home and it is the same here. When someone comes for a job here one of the questions we ask is "Are you a Mum?" If the answer is yes, that's half the battle as far as we are concerned. She knows what is expected of her.'

8.0 p.m.

Doreen comes out, followed by her friends, puts her arms round Judy and tells her she likes her. 'She always does that when it is time for her cigarette,' Judy says. Doreen is the only smoker among the residents and she is rationed strictly. She goes off out into the yard when Judy lights the cigarette. She is not allowed to smoke inside.

Judy is obviously liked by the residents – she comes in for a lot of thugs, from the women and the men. She laughs at the suggestion that they might call her Mum, too. 'I see myself as just one of the staff, and I'm Judy to the residents. Housemother sounds too grand a title for me. I've never had to take full responsibility for the whole place in my six months here. Mrs S is always a shout away in an emergency. The idea of being alone terrifies me.'

She is another one who took a strange route to her job – from nuclear physics via a spell of globe-trotting and a brief marriage, to bookselling and a job as a traffic warden. Working with the handicapped was simply something that had always appealed to her. 'They are like children really, the residents. Only when they have temper tantrums they are harder to contain than a six-year-old.'

The hardest part of the job, she admits, was getting used to people staring when she and another staff member took a group to the local pub in the evening. 'You could see them trying to work out who was staff and who was a resident. But you stop noticing the looks. In fact the people round here are mostly very nice to us. But when we took them to Blackpool, on holiday, it was awful. I've never met such open hostility.'

Doreen and entourage have returned from her smoking trip. She wants to talk about her new dress, bought for the society's annual dinner next week. They have a novel way of dealing with the business of clothes at the Home. Each resident's wardrobe is looked after by a member of the society. Two or three times a year, he or she comes in and goes through the clothes, checking to see what new items are needed. Then they take the resident out to buy them. Everyone has their own clothing, down to underwear. ('They actually share pants in some Local Authority places,' Mr H said with horror) and laundry is a duty of the housemothers.

8.15 p.m.

Mr H's school-teacher daughter leaves. She has popped in to mow the lawn. It is not an elaborate piece of garden, but fairly large. Nobody is employed to deal with it. Whichever member of staff or volunteer is free lends a hand. Judy, something of an enthusiast, has made herself responsible for the garden at the back of the Council house, growing fruit and vegetables, even tackling a tomato crop.

On the previous evening, Mr H's daughter had been in charge of the Gateway Club in the hall, ambitiously tackling rehearsals for the Society's version of *The Wizard of Oz* with some of the residents in the cast as well as some outsiders.

SANDFIELDS – BRINGING IN THE PROFESSIONALS

Hindley Home is one way for parents to run their own Home or hostel, pretty successfully. There are others – and the comparison in the style of running them is fascinating.

Some parent groups have raised the money, bought houses and furnished them, then handed over the running, staffing and selection of residents to the Social Services. They retain, by a sort of gentleman's agreement, a say in the running.

Another group has involved the Social Services from the planning stage, co-opting two social workers on to the building and management committees, acquiring a central government grant for the first four years to boost fund-raising, with the likelihood of further subsidizing in the future. A practical move, this – not only from a financial viewpoint, but because it is useful to have professional expertise, whilst retaining autonomy as a group.

But, as far as the lives of the children or adults who will live there are affected, the biggest question mark hangs over whether to employ an unqualified 'mumsy' figure to act as resident housemother and let the society members do the administering, or to turn it into a professionally run set-up.

Sandfields, twenty miles from Hindley Home, is very much the latter, but initially it was run by an unqualified middle-aged couple with a mentally handicapped daughter and with very much the same philosophy as at Hindley.

The system failed, for a variety of reasons. And two years ago the committee called in a professional administrator, with a background in mental health care, and his wife, a qualified nurse, to act as matron.

The couple, in their thirties, with a young family, live out. They were given *carte blanche* to get the place in order, though Mr K, the administrator, admits there were a few objections when he asked for the number of staff he felt necessary. Staffing was the first big problem, he says. When he came, there was a housemother, a part-time seamstress and part-time cook. Nobody else – though there had been a gardener and the four acres of ground were, as they still are, in stunningly well-kept order.

'It was just ticking over,' Mr K said. 'They shopped in the town, just like a housewife and the milkman called – but you cannot do that when you are catering for eighteen residents. Having a pair of trousers made in a shop for one of the residents – many of them are not standard sizes – was costing £25.

'My first three months were spent talking to people about contracts, arranging to have everything delivered at trade prices. Even clothing. I found a supplier who could make up the same trousers I mentioned for £8. We buy clothes in bulk (but in different styles) for economy, but one item each season is left for the resident to go out and buy with a staff member – to give the feeling of having something special and individual.'

Residents' beds were upped to twenty-six, including four short-stay, and two for emergencies; and the Borough Council were encouraged to treat the Home as part of their resources. The staff was increased to hitherto unknown levels: an administrator, a matron with a deputy and assistant plus a senior housemother making up the senior staff.

Under them are four full-time housemothers, two full-time

gardeners, three part-time domestics, two part-time cooks, and one part-timer each in the laundry and as a seamstress.

It guarantees parity in wages and conditions with Local Authority establishments, with a forty-hour week and an eight-hour day. This in turn guarantees continuity of staff and no dramatic turnover, Mr K says. Staff in general live out to give them a real break when off-duty, with one junior staff member sleeping in on rota every night and one senior member on call.

There is a GP in close contact – one of his first jobs was to put the residents on diets – and a psychiatrist from a nearby mental handicap hospital is on hand when needed.

It is highly efficient, with a turnover of £50,000 a year – yet the cost per resident per week is £48, slightly less than Hindley Home. Due, presumably, to good management.

How does it all affect the residents? Perhaps some of them preferred the old days when the shopping was done in the nearby town and they lived on unsupervised diets, like the rest of us. That, after all, is more in the 'ordinary lives in the community' mould.

I can only report having seen the Home run both ways and preferred the latter. However unhomely the forty-hour week sounds on paper, the staff are caring, informed and likeable. Perhaps it is easier to be those things when you get a decent wage and a fair time off.

The housemothers are not all qualified because Mr K, from his hospital experience, is convinced that the higher academic ability demanded for nursing training often keeps the best 'carers' out. But the competitive wage means they are not limited to school-leavers like other private places.

He gets down to the nitty-gritty in interviews with prospective staff – the sort of earthy areas that can make or break a good housemother. Will she mind cleaning dirty bottoms? How will she react if one of the men, whom she will have to deal with on the fairly intimate level of helping him to bath and dress, is sexually attracted to her? How is she going to cope with the couple of residents who cuddle continually in the common lounge?

All young female residents are on the pill on the 'better to be safe than sorry' principle. But, he says, echoing many other people in similar positions, relationships rarely progress beyond the cuddling-on-the-settee stage, embarrassing though that can be to everyone else sometimes.

Sandfields itself is a beautiful old house. 'We are half-way there with a house like this, instead of a purpose-built place. It is much more homely,' Mr K insists. Yet, the very layout prohibits some of the homelier freedoms. Sleeping areas are a few double rooms and two large dormitories, so it is not feasible for residents to come and go between their bedrooms and downstairs at any time of the day. Nor is there much privacy. The rooms and dormitories used to be done out in all one colour, matching carpets, curtains, bedspreads and walls and named accordingly – 'The Blue Room', etc.

Mr K is practically paranoid about the institutional suggestions of such conformity, however good it looks (they do it like this at Hindley Home) and has changed carpets and bedspreads, purely to bring in colours that do not match.

There is a big lounge downstairs, to accommodate everyone, but because there are now a percentage of older people, a smaller room is being converted into a quiet lounge for them, with their own television and tea-making facilities. The dining-room opens off a big kitchen, in which there appears to be an amazing number of staff accumulated. When the new régime moved in, all the kitchen appliances were of a domestic size. They have since been replaced with catering-size equipment, and money-saving schemes have been started. For instance, residents take packed lunches to their Adult Centres because of the big cost of lunches there. They then have a substantial main meal in the evening.

Like Hindley Home, the residents clock up record numbers of pantomimes and shows, amateur and professional. They get invited to local functions and youth clubs, though they are in the countryside, some distance from a classy residential area.

They, too, are pioneers. Like Hindley where residents have been introduced to swimming, people from Sandfields have taken up sailing. Holidays have been more imaginative – the last was on board two narrow boats. But then they are situated near a canal.

Both places tend to reject applicants who are not able to keep up the pace of the majority or disrupt group activities. Sandfields, though, abhors the idea of hauling parents and child 'before a selection panel of old biddies' and visits them at home, armed first with doctors' reports and histories. They have a trial period and, even so, admit to mistakes. They have one difficult young lady now, who has not settled, but she has been accepted and will stay.

Having heard strong talk of their differences, I was as much struck by the similarities. Mr H easily slips into the role of Mr K. Mrs S the 'Mum' does very much the same tasks as Mrs K the matron – and they both have similar backgrounds and training. It is not the attitude to residents that is different so much as the attitude to staff.

Sandfields has regular organized staff meetings and a recognizable hierarchy. At Hindley it is very informal and, as Mrs S put it as her assistant came in from the gardening to organize the ironing and do the baking. 'Over there, they have a person for every job. Here we all do everything'.

The Hindley Home system, while it works, is fine, but without the people who make it work it could break down badly. It seems inevitable that time, changes and expansion will force it eventually to opt for Sandfields' methods. That is not bad – just different.

The Future

Talk to parents about the kind of Home they would choose for their child should the need arise and, allowing for variation between the knowledgeable and the uninformed, the old-fashioned and the trendy, a pretty standard picture emerges.

It must be small, 'homely', not too far from home for visiting, welcoming to families; and it must have a high staff ratio of people who like and care deeply about their charges.

Nobody specifies whether this Home should be run by a Local Authority or the National Health Service. Nor do they get emotional about whether a new, specially trained profession should staff it, instead of traditionally trained nurses. It is irrelevant whether they have a string of letters propping up their names or not a single paper qualification – so long as they have the interest, intelligence and information to understand and care for their children mentally, physically and emotionally; and the sense to call in someone who knows the answers when they don't.

Rarely, either, is location a bone of contention. It matters not all that much whether the building is situated on the busiest street in town or in the middle of a field, providing the residents are neither plunged into situations they cannot cope with nor shut away.

The who-runs-what problem, the controversy over which training and which title should be held by the professionals who look after the mentally handicapped, the integration-versus-segregation issue: however hotly debated, these are internal problems. Only a few parents really care.

Simplistic it may be, but they find it hard to understand why the bureaucrats and professionals spend so much time talking, instead of putting the needs of the handicapped first and getting on with the caring.

There is room for hospital administered and based care; for Social Services neighbourhood units and independent and sheltered housing; for self-contained sheltered communities and small voluntary homes; for isolated and integrated communities and for joint projects – so long as they are each good of their kind.

Nobody queries the integrity and sense of a non-handicapped person who chooses to live in a remote village against someone who prefers life in a city flat. So why should there be only one route to perfect residential care for the mentally handicapped? People are infinitely varied, the mentally handicapped even more so. Conformity is not the answer. They and their families need choice.

At the moment they do not get much choice, because most parents, given the chance, opt for a similar type of care and there is not enough to go round. There are, in fact, not enough places of any kind, and the current trend towards encouraging families to keep their children at home overestimates the percentage who will manage to do so.

Initially, then, we need more residential units, with the needs and the preferences of the consumers – parents and the mentally handicapped themselves where possible – dictating the form and the percentage of each type. Parents must be given the right to choose. There are some occasions when they do know best. This is one.

What about the future? What I have covered are the standard types of residential accommodation, the bread and butter of long restay. It is obvious, though, that many people in this field are rethinking old 'facts', refusing to accept that the tried and traditional ways of accommodation for the mentally handicapped are the only ways. They are doing it *their* way. It is this sense of awareness that is the most heartening.

Some of the new ideas are just bright variations on an accepted theme; others are radical enough to be termed, as in medicine, 'fringe' care. Two of the best innovations – trend-setters that others could, should and probably will follow – concern children, the most vulnerable of all groups.

FIELD END HOUSE is a small, residential unit in the grounds of a disused London hospital, set up by courtesy of 'joint funding'. It caters for multiply handicapped children only, that unplaceable minority, which makes it unusual. Parental involvement, in management and handling the children, is a condition of acceptance, which probably makes it unique. Both factors, taken together, certainly make it noteworthy.

In fact the unit – for six permanent children and approximately twenty-four families within the Borough who can use it on a flexible day or short-term basis – is the result of parental pressure. Unusually, the pressure came from a group of parents whose children already had residential places but in hospitals far enough away to make visiting difficult. They wanted local provision and, not surprisingly, nothing remotely suitable for such severely handicapped children existed.

The finished unit must seem like a dream come true to the families, used to the official view that only hospitals could cope with their children's needs. Not that they have any insurmountable needs – just that they have to be carried and fed and are incontinent and some have fits: problems families cope with at home daily.

The outside surroundings are distinctly drab, but much money and initiative has been spent on transforming this ground floor corner of the old hospital into a large, well-equipped playroom, one- and two-bedded rooms and bathing and shower facilities. Parents are encouraged to come in when they wish to feed, bath and put their children to bed. It is their unit, too.

The staff ratio is very high – a superintendent with deputy and assistant plus eleven care officers on the caring side, to give cover for twenty-four-hour waking duty. They come from varied backgrounds. Of two I met, one was a teacher, one an ex-jazz musician.

With a short training course, they are expected to work on their own initiative and as part of a small team. Staff are split into teams, and each child is allocated to one team, responsible for his or her development and well-being. And they do put a lot of effort into playing with and 'stimulating' the children and seeing they are comfortable – perhaps because they are not rushed off their feet or because the interest and involvement of families is encouraging, or just because it is all so new. It had only been open a few months when I saw it. Whatever the reason, it was nice to see staff neither jaded, unimaginative or too busy to care. And with such traditionally unrewarding children, too.

Field End House was the result of three factors found in the same place at the same time. An Area Health Authority with an empty hospital, a Social Services Department with a duty to fulfil, and a group of parents who knew exactly what they wanted and fought for it. These parents are now part of the joint management team, which includes representatives from The Departments of Health, Social Services and Education (the children go out to local Special Schools).

There is a second unit opening upstairs in the same building, to be staffed and run independently. This will cater for the other 'untouchables' that the usual homes and hostels reject – the children who are hyperactive, difficult or psychotic. You can choose your own label.

If one authority can do it, surely the others – with the added guarantee of seeing it works – can manage it too.

PARENTS FOR CHILDREN* is a small adoption agency doing the impossible. At least, that is what we could have considered it a few years ago. With a DHSS grant, four dedicated social workers and a lot of faith, it is placing mentally handicapped children in permanent, adoptive homes.

Adoption, you notice, *not* fostering. They are not so keen on that, because, they say, it leaves the new families with less sense of commitment when the going gets rough. They are more likely to give up. But to digress – fostering is becoming an increasingly favoured way of finding homes for children.

One Local Authority I know of has a policy of never placing mentally handicapped children under the age of seven in Children's Homes. All go to foster parents, and they have a good success rate. It is another idea to be considered and enlarged and – as a few adventurous Authorities have done – tried out with teenagers and adults.

But back to PARENTS FOR CHILDREN, which flourished as a result of the shortage of healthy young babies placed for adoption. Prospective adopters have had to think twice about the possibilities and some, with information and guidance, have decided that they would enjoy bringing up a mentally handicapped child.

It is a fairly startling idea, and the agency has used sometimes controversial methods to make known the existence of these hard-to-place children on their books. They have publicized them, as individuals, in magazines and on radio and television. They have advertised them, with pictures and case histories, in a specialist magazine.

The right parents have been found largely by ignoring the rules about 'suitable' adopters, who must be of a certain age, status and religion. 'We believe,' said a social worker, 'that nobody is the perfect parent for every child, but that everyone is the right parent for *some* child.'

Successful adoptive parents here tend to be self-selecting. Many

*Parents for Children is at 22 Camden High Street, London NW1.

enquirers drop out during the early, informal discussion stages. It is expected.

The agency has placed a multiply handicapped eight-year-old – 'a little wild vegetable' – with a single woman; a brain-damaged girl with a family of older children; and several Down's Syndrome babies and toddlers with childless couples and families of all descriptions.

The obvious argument against adoption and fostering is that you are simply moving the problems that necessitated the original family asking for residential care on to another family's doorstep. Soon they, too, will come up against the same snags, with the same result.

On the face of it, yes. But the adoptive families, unlike natural parents, are volunteering for the role and are prepared. From this agency, at least, they get more follow-up support than natural parents – and the reassurance that no more is expected of them than of the original family. At some stage they, too, may need to send their child away from home. It is a decision they have to be prepared for.

The director of PARENTS FOR CHILDREN, Phillida Sawbridge, is convinced that if this happens even after a few years, these children who have no contact with their natural parents, will have gained from life in a family. They will always have a family to care about them and to visit and take them out. And that is looking at the worst that can happen.

This agency is, of course, a drop in the ocean. Local Authority adoption services could follow suit, but they would need much more time and staff and, above all, a change of attitude towards both the mentally handicapped and adoption. Wouldn't it be worth it, though? Look what at least a few children would gain.

Books and Papers Mentioned in the Text

Pauline Morris, *Put Away: Sociological Study of Institutions for the Mentally Retarded* (London, Routledge & Kegan Paul, 1969)

DHSS, *Better Services for the Mentally Handicapped* (London, HMSO, 1971)

Maureen Oswin, *Children Living in Long Stay Hospitals* (Spastics International Medical Publications, 1978)

NSMHC, *Directory of Residential Accommodation in England, Wales and Northern Ireland* (London, Nat. Soc. for Mentally Handicapped Children)

D. G. and D. M. Race, 'Investigation into the Effects of Different Caring Environments on the Social Competence of Mentally Handicapped Adults'. Progress Report No 1 (April 1975); Progress Report No 2 (April 1976). (Department of Applied Statistics, Reading University). These include a report of life at The Cherries.

Index